ISBN : 1912969416

CHAPTER 1 – F

'Don't expect perfect results overnight. Setting achievable goals and celebrating small successes can keep you motivated.'

Cellular Training

THERE IS A lot of research on the rebounder, or mini-trampoline, and why it is one of the best things for our overall health that we should have in our homes. In 1979, the *Journal of Applied Physiology* said jumping on a trampoline causes more biochemical changes than running. So, NASA's Biomechanical Research Division checked this out by comparing running, jogging, walking on a treadmill, and jumping – four different ways to work out.

When running on a treadmill, the back and head feel twice as much g-force as when jumping on a trampoline. That means that jumping doesn't put extra stress on the body, the heart doesn't have to work as hard, and you use up to twice as much oxygen as when you jog, run, walk, or run on a treadmill.

When you bounce, your g-force goes away at the top of the bounce. It means that you don't have any weight for a split second. At the bottom of the bounce, the g-force doubles, putting enough stress on your cells to make them change. Your body's 75 trillion cells move about 100 times a minute because of vertical acceleration and deceleration. Your cells can release more toxins and are less likely to break down. It is a great way to prevent degenerative diseases and slow the ageing process, and who doesn't want that?

Jumping also improves the flow of lymph. Since the lymphatic system doesn't have any chambers or pumps like the cardiovascular system, the body must move its muscles to move lymph fluid through the lymphatic system. When you jump, you speed up the rate at which your body gets rid of waste, which is a great way to eliminate toxins. Jumping helps stretch and strengthen the myofascial layers that cover your muscles and make them stronger, and combining these processes makes cellulite look less noticeable.

Training on a rebounder will also benefit the bones and help to prevent and treat osteoporosis. Because jumping is low-impact training, muscles and bones don't sustain the damage caused by high-impact exercise, so the cells of every bone in your body get more minerals and blood flow. It is commonly known that NASA found their astronauts lost about 20% of their bone density while in space because they were weightless. NASA studied rebounding and found it an effective way to increase bone density again.

The 'fun' benefits of rebounding cannot be over-emphasised, and it is a form of 'stress rejection'. After just one session, the body can feel more relaxed for up to 90–120 minutes. It helps you sleep better and lifts your mood. Now, here's the thing: you can't jump on a trampoline without smiling at least once. It's a reflex, like how women open their mouths when they put on mascara or how we yawn when someone else yawns. When you jump on a trampoline, you can't help but smile. It is just not possible. It is safe for all body types, so no matter how heavy you are or how bad your health is, you can jump on a trampoline in different ways to get all the health benefits without putting stress on your body.

TAKEAWAY

JUMPGA cellular training. You'll be amazed at how you can strengthen and stretch your body, eliminate toxins, and improve the appearance of your skin. Consider getting access to a rebounder in the gym or at home, knowing it takes only a short workout (see Chapter 5) to reap the benefits.

Midlife MOT

THERE HAS NEVER been a time when I thought exercise was optional. Getting fit is not a one-off event. It's a process, a series of small movements and slight adjustments. Those small changes can ultimately get you from where you are now to where you want to be. Take the simple test below to gauge where you are now.

1. What's your resting heart rate?

Your MOT starts with your heart, the only muscle in your body that has to function 24 hours a day, seven days a week. 'Heart rate is a simple metric of fitness,' Dr Rankin explains. 'If your heart is beating as you walk up the stairs, you're in trouble.' Your resting heart rate determines the efficiency of the organ. If you're a serious athlete, you should aim for a heart rate of 60-100 beats per minute (bpm) or 40-60 beats per minute (bpm). If your heart rate falls outside those ranges, see your doctor before attempting tests 4 through 9 on this page.

2. Can you blow out a match six inches away?

The Snider Test is a primitive method of determining lung function, albeit superseded by more precise tests accessible at doctors' offices or through internet kits. If you cannot extinguish the match, you should seek medical assistance.

3. String test

A group of British academics examined the health of 300,000 adults in 2012. The researchers discovered that the height-to-weight ratio could help predict heart attacks and strokes. high blood pressure, cardio-vascular events and diabetes. 'Waist circumference has to be less than half your height to help everyone in the world live longer,' said Dr Margaret Ashwell, the study's lead author. Cut a length of string to your height from head to toe, divide it in half, and see if it wraps around your waist one inch above your belly button.

4. Step test

The Step Test assesses an individual's aerobic fitness. Participants step up and down, on and off, an aerobics-style step for THREE minutes to raise heart rate and evaluate the heart's recovery rate in the minute after the step test.

5. How long can you hold a plank position?

The plank is a great way to measure your core strength, essential for your posture (see tests 10 and 11). Lie face down on the floor, elbows tucked in at your sides and hands beside your shoulders. Raise yourself to the point where your forearms and toes are the only parts of your body that contact the ground with your shoulders directly above your elbows.

Males and females: Poor = 45 seconds or less; average = 45-75 seconds; good = 75-120 seconds; exceptional = more than 120 seconds.

6. How long can you stand on one leg with your eyes closed?

Proprioception is the ability to tell where your body is in space even while your eyes are closed. And this is where flexibility comes into play. The single-leg balance test will immediately reveal your proprioception's quality. You should be able to hold your position for at least five seconds without opening your eyes or placing your leg down. You're doing well if you can get up to 20 seconds.

7. Flexibility

The sit and reach test assesses your hamstrings, hips, and lower back flexibility. It's a decent gauge of your overall flexibility. Your flexibility is functional if you can reach your soles. A good result for a 50-year-old lady would be 19 inches or 16.5 inches for a guy.

8. Physical exertion test

High-intensity exercises to push your heart rate and find out how long it can stay there while maintaining your strength and power. Burpees is a total body workout. Start with a plank, then swing your hips forward on the way up, so your feet fall flat on the ground. Jump as high as you can while pointing your arms towards the ceiling. It should be a dynamic movement that is both smooth and rapid. A good result is five; over 12 is impressive.

9. How good is your posture?

Stand up and look down at your feet for the lower part of your body. What direction are your toes pointing? Your feet should be facing forward so that your legs and hips work equally. Lean against a wall, lightly contacting the wall with your heels. What is the distance between your head and the wall? The balance of your body determines your posture; if your body is balanced, your head will be contacting the wall. Your lower back and bum will benefit as well.

10. Elastic band

Reinforcing your intentions needs an anchor (a stimulus-response pattern) that can help you consciously retrigger positive associations. The '*rubber-band* technique' is an external trigger for an internal response to your desire. When you find yourself wavering from your goal, you snap the rubber band on your wrist to re-access and reinforce your intention.

TAKEAWAY

Before you start the training, why not take this physical MOT? Not doing this simple test will defeat the programme. Because if you don't know where you are going, how will you know when you get there?

Do You Need a Better Balance?

CAN YOU STAND on one leg for ten seconds? Scientists say you're twice as likely to die early if you can't stand on one leg like a flamingo when you're in your 60s. Authors of a study in the *British Journal of Sports Medicine* say that middle-aged people who can't stand on one leg are twice as likely to die young.

Researchers in Brazil looked at 2,000 people between 50 and 75 and found that those who couldn't stand on one leg for 10 seconds were 84% more likely to die in the next ten years.

Another study of people in their fifties found that those who could stand on one leg for ten seconds with their eyes closed were most likely to be healthy and fit in 13 years. Those who only got two seconds were three times as likely to die before they turned 66.

People with heart disease, high blood pressure, or diabetes are more likely to have trouble keeping their balance during the 'simple and safe' balance test.

The team said that the 'flamingo test' could be used in regular health checks for older people to give 'useful information' about their risk of dying. Unlike aerobic fitness, muscle strength, and flexibility, the balance stays pretty good until a person is in their sixties, when it worsens.

But new evidence shows that it can also be a sign that something terrible will happen. Even in otherwise healthy adults, being unable to stand on one leg for 20 seconds or more has been linked to a higher risk of damage to small blood vessels in the brain, decreased cognitive function, and stroke. Some researchers have also found a strong link between poor balance and the number of cases of dementia.

According to the researchers, balance checks aren't usually part of health checks for older people because there isn't a standard way to measure them. There is also not much information about how balance affects health other than that it makes you more likely to trip and fall.

As we get older, our balance will always get worse in some ways. In our twenties and thirties, we each have about 70,000 specialised nerve cells called motor neurons in the lower part of our spinal cords. These neurons connect with our trunk and leg muscles to control our balance and movement. Our ability to stay balanced depends on the nervous system telling the muscles to contract and the body to move into place and on the muscles being able to send information back to the brain. It's a never-ending feedback loop that works less well as we age.

For the study, which started in 1994, 1,702 people in Brazil were asked to take different fitness tests, such as standing on one leg for 10 seconds without holding on to anything.

So that everyone did it the same way they put the front of one foot on the back of the other lower leg, kept their arms at their sides, and looked straight ahead.

Researchers also noted how much they weighed, how big their waists were, and their blood pressure. On average, the volunteers were watched for seven years.

The rate went up with age. Only 5% of people ages 51 to 55 failed the task, but 54% of people ages 71 to 75 did not pass. During the study, about 123 people died. Scientists didn't find any apparent differences in how people died between those who could finish the test and those who couldn't.

After considering age, gender, and health problems, those who couldn't stand on one leg without help for 10 seconds were 84% more likely to die from any cause in the next ten years. Most people who failed the test were also in worse health. A more significant number of them were overweight, had heart disease, high blood pressure, or had bad blood fat profiles. And there were three times as many people with type 2 diabetes in this group.

The researchers said that all the people who took part were white Brazilians, so the results might not be accurate for people of other races or from different countries. And there was no information about things that could affect balance, like whether or not the volunteers had fallen recently, how active they were, what they ate, if they smoked, or if they used drugs.

Standing on one leg while you brush your teeth takes you off-balance to balance. And balancing on one leg helps to work your stabilising muscles – including your adductors (inner thigh muscles) and abductors (outer thigh muscles) which keep you steady on your feet. So, every time you brush your teeth shift your weight to one side and stand on a single leg with your morning brush. Then in the evening, balance on your left side.

TAKEAWAY

Single leg standing on a rebounder will challenge your balance to improve it. Five minutes of balance exercise produces a sensation that lasts far longer than the time spent exercising.

'Remember that everyone is different, and what works for one person may not work for another'

R & R (Rest & Recovery)

FITNESS RECOVERY IS essential, and you don't have to be a professional athlete to benefit from it. If you want to get leaner, fitter, and stronger, it's tempting to believe that the quickest approach to improving your fitness and body shape is to exercise hard every day. But what you do outside of the gym is just as essential as what you do inside the gym.

So, why is it so crucial?

Recovery isn't a new concept; it's the time it takes for the body to adjust to the stressors of exercise, restore energy supplies, and repair muscle tissue that has been damaged. We gain strength by causing slight tears in our muscle tissue during workouts. The body heals these tears during recovery, making them more resistant to future exercise. You'd continue to tear your muscle if you didn't recuperate, which might lead to harm.

There are further consequences to not healing correctly. If you don't use adequate recovery procedures, you may get sub-optimal effects from your training and slower growth. Lack of recovery can harm your immune system, making you susceptible to sickness, low mood and disturbed sleep.

It's vital to remember that you adapt and grow while you recuperate from your workout, not during it. The issue for many people who prefer to push themselves isn't overtraining but rather a lack of recovery.

How much time do you need to relax and recover?

Average muscle recovery takes between 24 and 48 hours as a general guideline. Many people, especially those new to exercise, who have taken a lengthy break, or are starting a new training cycle, can have DOMS (delayed onset muscle soreness) for up to 48 hours after a hard workout. However, if the discomfort lasts for four to five days, you may be training with too much volume and intensity.

During rest and healing do not, however, simply do nothing. Yoga, foam rolling, or focusing on your post-workout nutrition are all examples of fitness recovery.

Nutrition is essential, and anyone who works out regularly should consume a high-protein diet. Protein's primary function in the body is to promote growth and repair, reducing muscular soreness following an exercise. Diets can help prevent inflammation by avoiding foods that cause the body to become inflamed.

Inflammation raises the danger of damage and the time it takes to heal. When minimising inflammation, eating a diet high in green vegetables and essential fats containing anti-inflammatory omega-3s, such as fatty salmon, while reducing overly-processed meals is an excellent rule.

Pro-inflammatory foods are refined sugar, alcohol, trans and hydrogenated fats, and pro-inflammatory omega-6 fats like seed and vegetable oils.

'Active recuperation' is another term for it

Even when you're recovering, staying active, moving your body, and working your muscles are critical. This is doing low-intensity exercise in between more strenuous workouts, which can help relieve pain by improving blood flow and nutrition delivery to sore areas.

A light walk, swim, bike ride, rebounding, or even yoga are examples of low-impact, non-overly strenuous active recuperation. Massage or foam rolling can help to improve circulation and nutrition delivery while also 'breaking down' tight muscles.

Due to the growing demand from gym-goers for recuperation options, studios are now offering specific programmes to help people. A 'stretch' class, for example, uses myofascial release techniques to relieve muscle tension. Some gyms have dedicated recovery lounges with equipment to speed up the healing process, such as compression stockings to improve circulation after a workout. Compressed air is used to massage limbs and mobilise fluid in the high-tech boots for the feet and legs.

Our gym clothing is getting in on the recharge game, with mineral-lined fabric that reflects infrared light to your body, thus speeding up muscle recovery.

But recovery isn't just for the physical; it's also vital for mental wellness. It's no accident that the number of franchise and independent relaxation and recuperation studios has increased. In recent years, the expansion of the health, fitness, and wellness business has been critical in encouraging people to sit up and pay more attention to recovery as part of a broader understanding of our health.

TAKEAWAY

No matter what training you do, working out hard all the time is a fast way to get tired and hurt. Workout fans often get stuck in a cycle of workout, rest, and workout. It might sound like a good thing, but working out isn't just to recover so you can work out again. It's to recover and then adapt to get stronger or perform better. When you're just starting to feel better and then go back to the gym, it's only a matter of time before your body says it's had enough and gives up.

*'Fitness can mean different things to different people.
It can involve anything from going for a walk or a
swim to lifting weights or doing yoga'*

Hand Grip Strength

'A SOUND MIND in a sound body' is a famous statement about the link between exercise and brain health. Exercise has been proved in numerous research projects to boost cognitive ability. Researchers are even using body strength to predict brain health in a new study showing that grip strength is a reliable indicator of one's mental health and can be used to detect problems before other symptoms appear. Yet as we age, we tend to get reduced hand circulation and often notice a feeling of stiffness in the fingers.

A basic gym routine is the most obvious answer to preserving your strength. It should include various forms of weight training and sit-ups – but everything can impact your strength.

Wrist Strength

A firm handshake in business is essential. Experts believe the decline in grip power is part of the overall loss of muscle strength, which starts in our 40s and accelerates in our 70s. We lose between 3 and 5 percent of muscle mass per decade.

Weakening grip strength has been associated with an overall loss of power and can provide valuable insight into an individual's risk of future disease. The *Journal of Alzheimer's Disease* found poor grip was a sign of cognitive impairment, which leads to dementia.

Each 5kg reduction in grip strength – for reference, a 30-year-old man has a grip strength of about 40kg on average – was associated with an 18 percent greater chance of severe cognitive impairment.

A US study in the journal *Clinical Interventions in Ageing* concluded that grip strength is a predictive marker of bone density, fractures, falls, cognition, depression, sleep and mortality.

You never see gym-goers exercising to maintain grip strength; instead, they focus on superficial muscles to look good. This means your grip can become neglected, and you will only realise it has deteriorated when it affects your day-to-day life, such as when you struggle to open jars or you lift something awkwardly.

A seemingly simple manoeuvre like gripping is a very complex action. It involves two muscles that run from the forearm across the wrist into the fingers, called the superficial and the profundus (these help us flex our fingers) and smaller muscles inside the hand that stabilise the wrist joint and help with dexterity.

When we grip something, all these muscles shorten, pulling the fingers into the palm while holding the wrist in a fixed position, so it doesn't move. Just like other muscles in our body, if we don't exercise those in our arms and hands that control grip strength, they can quickly decline.

The ability to grip is one reason humans have been so successful. Our grip sets us apart from other mammals because we can use our thumb to hold tools, for instance. Losing the ability to use our thumb removes about 75% of the function of the whole arm.

Medical conditions such as arthritis, diabetes and trapped nerves can also affect our grip strength. It's a case of 'use it or lose it'. If you want to retain your grip strength, regular exercise is one way.

Handgrip exercise has the following advantages:

1. **Builds forearm strength** – Training using a tennis ball can improve your forearm circumference, leading to more muscular arms.

2. **Helps to avoid injuries** – Grip strength workouts tone your hands and forearms, lowering your chance of injury while participating in activities such as tennis and weightlifting.

3. **Strengthens your hands** – Handgrip exercise, without a doubt, contributes to increasing hand endurance. It increases the resistance on your hand, which forces you to apply power to grow muscle and strength.

4. **Provides greater dexterity** – Handgrip training also helps develop agility by allowing fingers to grow independently.

It doesn't matter how big your biceps are or how much you can bench press. If your fingers are weak – you lack grip strength.

TAKEAWAY

Your grip can also tell a lot about how healthy you are. A study published in the Journal of Strength and Conditioning Research *found that grip strength predicts muscular endurance and overall strength. Other studies have shown that having a firmer grip is linked to a lower chance of having a heart attack or stroke. Researchers say the results indicate a link between a healthy heart and strong muscles.*

Lean Torso at Any Age

IT TAKES WORK to have defined abs as you get older. I know people who train regularly, and for neither love nor money, they have yet to achieve a six-pack. And it gets harder through midlife because you lose muscle mass causing your metabolism to slow down; your body becomes less efficient at turning food into energy.

This is what causes the well-known 'middle-aged spread'. It happens to many people after 40, even if their lifestyle and diet don't change.

As well as building muscle, losing extra weight during midlife becomes more challenging. The sex hormones, especially testosterone, decline with age, along with human growth hormone (HGH), making it much harder to lose weight and gain muscle. Women have it worse with their suite of health issues relating to reduced levels of oestrogen and progesterone.

Men can have up to 30% more body fat than they did in their 20s by the time they are in their 60s and 70s. Compared to women, who naturally have a distribution of primarily subcutaneous fat, which accumulates under the skin, especially in the gluteal area, men are more prone to gain visceral fat over the belly and inside their abdominal cavity, surrounding their internal organs.

At 65, I'm not as taut as I was in my twenties, but I still prefer 'lean' over 'bulk'. My body fat percentage is in the 10% – 14% range, which is sustainable for people who exercise regularly. A lean body muscle mass (low body fat with visible muscular definition) can help protect against bones losing their density as you age. Osteoporosis and frailty in later life can put you at significant risk as they lead to falls and fractures.

Building strength is empowering. That is why the internet is awash with midlifers posting pictures of their muscles. Everyone wants to be strong and getting visible abs, but it is very challenging and needs a lot of commitment, so it becomes a badge of honour. The abs are there; we all have them, but you must put yourself in a sustained, focused health and fitness programme to see them. As ever, with everything regarding bodywork with age, you need to allow a reasonable timeframe to achieve a lean body because it does take time. Realistically, it can take twelve months to lose a significant amount of body fat safely.

I taught my first fitness class over 40 years ago and I have witnessed how my body's composition has changed with age. What I did in my 20s does not work in my 60s. Midlifers are living longer, and with over one billion people now at 60 +, trainers need a more specific approach to age-related fitness.

The government recommends that people exercise for 150 minutes per week doing moderate-intensity activity. That's about 30 minutes a day just walking on a treadmill five times a week. It should be more like a minimum of 60 minutes of daily exercise, and you can achieve this by putting more energy into everything you do.

However, not everyone achieves that level. Instead, people have become more sedentary, with a significant drop-off in physical activity levels, especially as they age, or for those looking for an exercise strategy that requires as little time as possible – hence, the rise of short, high-intensity interval training programmes.

The first step to defining your abs must start with fat loss – nutrition. The second step is to see exercise as not a way to lose weight but to improve your well-being.

Eat right, train smart and the ideal body composition (those defined abs) will be achievable by following my full-body exercise programme which encompass the five components of physical fitness: cardiovascular endurance, flexibility, mobility, muscular strength, and endurance.

I focus on developing a more efficient body that is less prone to the mechanical ravages of ageing, training the body as a whole. There is an emphasis on the trunk region because it is the most critical part of your body and can be harder to train than other parts.

TAKEAWAY

You don't have to make significant changes to get fit, lean, and defined. All you must do is do the right kind of exercise, as opposed to punishing your body with excessive overload, or trying to get away with the bare minimum. My programme is a form of exercise that will not only slow the ageing process but will also provide you with the highly coveted 'six-pack'.

CHAPTER 2 – HEALING

'Make healthier choices when it comes to what you put into your body'

Allergies and Your Gut

DID YOU KNOW that the majority of the cells in your body are not human? They are microbes. They are made up of bacteria, viruses, and fungi, mostly living in your gut.

Microbes help you digest food, produce important vitamins, and stimulate your immune system. They also help fight off pathogens and can change your mood, metabolism, and appetite.

The microbiota in your gut, skin allergies and a protein that protects against viral infections are all connected. Researchers have found that a broken immune system can change the gut microbiota, which can cause severe allergic skin reactions.

Your face shows what's inside you. If your face or skin turns red, feels burning hot, or gets very itchy suddenly, chances are you're allergic to something. You've probably tried everything to get rid of that annoying rash. Have you thought it may have something to do with how you feel or something you've eaten?

Scientists have previously found that gut bacteria are linked to allergic reactions. A new study led by two scientists from the French National Centre for Scientific Research (CNRS) found that skin allergies can be caused by problems with the immune system, which change the makeup of the gut microbiota.

If a virus-detecting protein isn't in your gut, things could get nasty. Scientists used mice that didn't have a protein called MAVS, so they could study the link between the immune system, allergies, and gut bacteria. The immune system uses this protein to determine if a virus is in the body. When they looked at the bacteria in the guts of these mice, they found that the bacteria had changed in a big way. The mice that didn't have good immune systems had almost 30 times more bacteria from the phylum Deferribacte'es and more Bacteroides vulgatus.

When the types of bacteria in the gut changed, the intestinal wall became more porous. It made it easy for certain gut bacteria to get to the spleen and lymph nodes through the bloodstream, which made the allergic reaction worse.

What stood out, though, was that the mice seemed to have severe allergic reactions on their skin. Could these two things have something to do with each other? To find out why the team gave the changed microbiota to normal mice and saw that the mice also had severe allergic reactions. That means that the transplanted gut bacteria were to blame.

One good thing about this study is that it opens the door to new, non-drug ways to treat skin allergies. Probiotics might be the way to go, especially if you have allergies. A review of 23 studies that looked at the effects of different probiotics on seasonal allergies showed that, compared to a placebo, most probiotics made allergy symptoms better.

For example, people with seasonal allergic rhinitis (hay fever) felt less sick when they took a strain of Bifidobacterium lactis. In another study, Lactobacillus acidophilus improved allergy symptoms just as much. However, most of these studies used different strains of bacteria, which makes it hard to draw firm conclusions.

Does this mean that probiotics will become the new way to treat allergies? There are still more questions to ask. First, we need to figure out which strains of bacteria are good for which allergy symptoms. Next, knowing which probiotics will work for each of us is essential. Everyone's gut, immune system, and skin microbiome are different, so it will take some time to figure out.

TAKEAWAY

The microbiota in your gut, skin allergies, and a protein that protects against viral infections are all connected. Researchers have found that a broken immune system can change the gut microbiota, which can cause severe allergic skin reactions. Support your skin in the best way possible by taking care of your body, and eat well.

'Remember that everyone is different, and what works for one person may not work for another'

Arthritic Athlete

FITNESS IS ASSOCIATED with challenging exercises rather than rehabilitation, stretching hamstrings and spatial awareness. With age comes wisdom. Exercise wisdom does not mean tedious exercise – it means training smarter, not harder.

I created Midlife Fitness as a recovery programme to strengthen my body following various surgeries and injuries. The most important lesson I learned is that there is no quick fix. I have spent years self-experimenting: I have trained with the like of Tatsuo Suzuki, the Japanese karateka who is instrumental in spreading the martial art of karate to Europe and the United States. I climbed a mountain and sat with a sage, travelled to India to practise yoga and explored many ancient disciplines to enable me to teach what I know to be the ultimate fix.

In the times we live in today, practices like yoga and meditation are essential components being incorporated into traditional training regimes to calm people down or increase their focus.

Researchers from Ulleval University Hospital in Norway report that people who use meditation after training reduce their production of lactate, the ache-inducing by-product of anaerobic exercise, and recover their fitness levels faster.

More people should do KUN-AQUA , which emphasises slow movement, static positions, and extension poses (see Chapter5 for more detail). These movements do not negatively impact concentration and body function and make it harder to hyper-extend joints. KUN-AQUA emphasises awareness and quality of movement – two significant components to living well.

Static poses in the water require the muscles to work hard to stabilise the body. Not only is core stability a foundation for movement, but being more stable allows you to increase your range of motion.

The great thing about KUN-AQUA is that it's performed at a slow pace. When walking or running outside, you don't have time to think about hip rotation, but you'll have all the time in the world to focus on body movement while doing KUN-AQUA. It can improve your kinaesthetic awareness, and that can improve your gait.

Again, the slow, controlled movements of KUN-AQUA allow you to detect muscular imbalances. Most people tend to have stronger muscles on one side of their body because we are generally left or right-sided. Those asymmetries can lead to injury if not corrected. KUN-AQUA can help.

I often meet middle-aged people with various aches and pains who quickly tell me why they cannot exercise. Although I suffer with chronic pain, exercise enables me to function and control the pain. My mother had arthritis and I am beginning to develop the disorder myself. I suppose that makes me an 'arthritic athlete'. I can't reverse my arthritis, but I am slowing down the progression of the disease and managing the condition. The KUN-AQUA exercise not only eases my pain but also helps me maintain and even improve my own self-awareness.

KUN-AQUA exercise avoids putting too much strain on the joints. The low impact exercises are a better option for people with arthritis. Also, there are not too many movements that twist the joints, which can increase the pain that arthritis causes. I have witnessed how this exercise effectively reduces pain and improves function and quality of life in clients with osteoarthritis.

Strengthening the muscles around the joints is an essential element of the treatment for osteoarthritis, as it helps to improve cartilage quality, nerve activation and coordination between muscles. Moreover, stronger muscles help the joints to absorb body weight while walking. Strong muscles facilitate the absorption and distribution of weight at the hip and knee joints, thereby increasing stability and improving function and mobility.

KUN-AQUA exercises are particularly beneficial for overweight and older patients with osteoarthritis. The waves and buoyancy of water support the body's weight, reducing the impacts on joints and the intensity of pain.

TAKEAWAY

The water's aqua static pressure helps relax the muscles, relieve stress, reduce muscle stiffness, and facilitate movement. Athletes who use KUN-AQUA exercises do so because they understand that it is the epitome of training smarter, not harder. So, if it is good enough for world-class athletes, it is good enough for you.

Death by Sitting

SITTING FOR LONG periods every day is terrible for our health. The effects are similar to those of smoking cigarettes. Researchers in the US now think our inactivity is a much bigger reason why health problems are worsening than what we eat.

Studies show that you can't undo the damage that sitting for long periods does just by working out regularly. One of these studies, published in the *Archives of Internal Medicine* which includes a whopping 220,000 people, took into account things like age, smoking status, weight, etc., and how much exercise people did. The study found that people who sit for more than 8 hours a day have a 15% higher chance of 'all-cause mortality' within three years than people who sit for less than 4 hours a day. For people who sit for 11 hours or more, that chance goes up to 40%. 'Long-term sitting is a risk factor for death from any cause, regardless of how much you move around'. They found that even physically fit people who spend a lot of time sitting down seem at a higher risk.

More and more people are using standing desks. While this is better than sitting for long periods of time, it doesn't completely solve the problem. It works some of your muscles, which is good, but it doesn't let you move as much as you need to, which is terrible. Remember that sitting is bad for your health, not because of how you sit, but because it keeps you from moving around. Your cardiovascular, muscular, and lymphatic systems don't work nearly enough when you stand to give your body the stimulation it needs. Also, standing for long periods has harmful effects, such as putting stress on the lower back, making you tired, swelling your legs, and making you more likely to get varicose veins.

A recent Australian study found that replacing two hours of sitting with standing didn't make much of a difference in blood sugar and cholesterol levels (2% lower), but moving around at a standing desk helped people lose weight (11% lower Body Mass Index), get slimmer (7.5

cm smaller waist), and lower their blood sugar and cholesterol levels by a lot. (October 14, 2015, *European Heart Journal*)

The best way to fight the harmful effects of sitting all day is to take short exercise breaks or do some physical activity at your desk. After 30 minutes of sitting, our metabolism slows by 90%, so we need to move our whole bodies at least once an hour. It keeps our bodies from going into hibernation mode and moves fat (triglycerides) and sugar (glucose) from our bloodstream to our muscles, where they can be burned off.

Short bursts of exercise throughout the day, like rebounding, doing 10 squats at your desk or press-ups against the wall can help you feel less tired, have more energy, and be in a better mood. In contrast to the effects of a single long bout of activity, the results of short bursts of activity last all day long.

Correct Sitting Position

- Straighten your back and put your shoulders back as you sit up. Your buttocks should be against the back of the chair.

- When sitting, the back should have all three normal curves. Using a small, rolled-up towel or a lumbar roll, you can keep your back's natural curves.

- Sit at the very end of your chair and completely slouch. Pull yourself up and make as much of the curve in your back as you can. Hold for a short time. Let go of the position a little (about 10 degrees). It is an excellent sitting posture.

- While sitting, put the same amount of weight on each hip.

- Make a right angle with your knees. Keep your knees about the same height as your hips or a bit higher. (If you need to, use a footrest or stool.) Don't put your legs together.

- Put your feet on the floor flat.

- Try not to stay in one place for more than 30 minutes.

- Change the height of your chair and workstation so you can sit close to your work and tilt it up towards you. Relax your shoulders and rest your elbows and arms on your chair or desk.

- Don't twist at the waist when sitting in a chair that rolls and turns. Turn your whole body instead.

- Move to the front of the chair before standing up. Stand up by putting your legs straight. Don't bend forward from the waist. Do ten standing backbends right away to stretch your back.

TAKEAWAY

A few minutes of regular 5-minutes exercise during the day will give you everything you need to fight back against the dangers of being inactive and improve your health and fitness. The benefits can last a lifetime.

Injury Free

AFTER YEARS OF not hitting the gym, you will need to return to working out gradually and safely if you want to avoid hurting yourself. The quickest path to an injury is to rush the process of returning to exercise, doing too much too soon. It can often lead to overuse syndromes or injuries like shin splints. The horrible news is it takes only a few weeks for you to lose muscle strength and some cardio fitness.

But the good news is that even after inactivity, your body is fantastic and will rebuild your strength and endurance. But listen to your body as you go – you will need to push it progressively for a gradual challenge.

Pay special attention to personal risk areas, such as damaged knees or a chronic back condition. Your age can affect your risk of injury, so you may need to modify your training programme to accommodate your changing physique.

Gender can also play a role in your body's distinct responses. Twist-and-turn actions in skiing, basketball, and racquet sports put women at a higher risk of injury. Workouts involving many planes of motion, such as yoga, stair-stepping machines, or cycling, on the other hand, may put men at risk of injury.

Small Steps

Don't expect to breeze right into the gym doing what you previously did. You are no longer in your best shape, and trying to prove otherwise will give you an injury on your first day back. Play it safe and start slowly with lower weights and less intensity. Training is a marathon, not a sprint; give yourself time to strengthen your body's connective tissues and increase the resistance capacity. With a thought-out conservative approach, you will provide your body the time it needs to adjust and adapt to the stresses you're placing upon it.

The First Two Weeks

The initial beginning phase is crucial as you start to work your entire body and re-train your neural pathways. Start with weights at least 50% lower than you used before. You can adjust this upward as things get easier. After four to six weeks, your body should be feeling a lot like its former self – a point when you can consider the transition to heavier weights.

Postural Alignment

On a day-to-day basis, people have poor postural alignment. Poor posture was made worse by people spending more time at home during the pandemic. Poor posture weakens your entire musculoskeletal structure. To combat this, stand tall; ensure you're not hunching over your screen/phone, and position it in a way that you're not straining to see it.

Warm-up

The way you move your body in the gym will be different to training at home, and you will recruit muscles you haven›t worked for a while. For this reason, it is essential to do a proper warm-up – preparing the muscles to get the blood flowing is necessary to avoid injury.

Smarter, not Harder

Always focus on quality over quantity. Ensure you maintain good posture and focus on complete movements rather than compromising your form for a higher number of repetitions or how many sets you do. There are no achievement badges for stupidity. Staying injury free is the key to a smooth transition back to the gym.

Never Assume

Don't be embarrassed if you've forgotten how to work the machines or set up the fixed weight apparatus. Gym Instructors are there for a reason – use them, and don't be ashamed to ask for a quick refresher. Consider going one step further and book in for a programme review to reset your gym confidence and techniques. Better still, book a personal training session.

Define your Objectives

It's critical to set goals when getting back into shape. Determining why you're going to the gym might aid in training planning and technique. A common cause of sporting injuries is

doing too much, too soon. Find the suitable activity and pace for your fitness level and work your way up. And avoid making the same moves too much.

R&R

Within a few weeks, you'll be right back to where you were before, but going too hard too early could result in pain or injury and set you back even further. To this end, rest and recovery is an essential phase on the road to peak fitness, so if you need a rest day, take it.

Listen to Your Body

We need to listen to our bodies sometimes, no matter how active or sedentary we are. In this fast-paced life, we often hurt our bodies to get fit, but we never really give our muscles a chance to recover. It is just as crucial to our workout routine as the exercises themselves, so ensure you're not hurting yourself more than you're helping.

TAKEAWAY

If you don't feel any effects the day after a workout, feel free to go back to it. If you feel tired or under the weather, just do yourself a favour and relax. And the best place to do this is at home, with your feet up. After all, we all need a little balance in our lives.

Osteoporosis

OSTEOPOROSIS IS A disease that weakens bones. About 3.5 million people in the UK and Ireland have it. It is common in women over 50 because oestrogen levels drop quickly after menopause. However, osteoporosis is also common in men and people who are more likely to get it because of their genes, taking certain medications like corticosteroids, or having illnesses like anorexia.

Every year it breaks 500,000 bones in the UK. It has a terrible effect on people's personal and financial lives. Clinicians at the Royal Osteoporosis Society (ROS) say that osteoporosis is a 'silent disease' because it is not known enough by the public.

The choices we make as we grow older can directly affect the health of our bones. By taking steps to improve bone health, we can avoid the painful effects of the condition in the future. The ROS know how easy it is to forget about our bones until they break. Here's why and how they want everyone to care for their bones.

1. You might not know you have it until it's too late

Osteoporosis has no symptoms, and often the first sign bones have lost strength is that they break easily after a minor bump or fall. People often think osteoporosis causes aches and pains, but this is not true. The condition itself doesn't hurt, but the pain that can come from breaking a bone is real.

2. It can make you lose your freedom

Fractures in the legs, hips, or spine can make it hard to move around in the short term, and breaks in the arms or wrists can make it hard to do everyday things. Broken bones not only hurt a lot and lower the quality of life in the short term, but they can also cause long-term disability and loss of independence.

3. It can change how tall you are

Many fractures from osteoporosis happen after a fall, but spinal fractures can occur without an apparent accident or injury and may not hurt. The ROS says broken bones in the back can become flattened or wedge-shaped and stay that way even after the bones have healed. It changes the shape of the spine.

4. Both work and life at home can be affected

The ROS says that osteoporosis fractures can make some people so sick or hurt that they can't work. Many people with osteoporosis say that their work or their partner's work is affected by the disease, making them cut their hours or retire early. People's hobbies and social lives are often affected, and some people cut back or stop doing these things, which makes them feel alone.

5. Weight can be important

The ROS says that your risk of osteoporosis and broken bones increases if you are underweight or overweight, so it's usually a good idea to keep your weight in a healthy range.

6. Working out lessens the chance of osteoporosis

The ROS says you can keep your bones strong by giving them work. The best way to do this is to combine weight-bearing exercises with impact and muscle-strengthening exercises. The first type involves being on your feet and putting an extra force or jolt through your bones. Do some Pilates, go walking, or rebounding. But avoid bending and twisting movements; they can put too much strain on the body.

7. Take vitamin D

The ROS says that people who don't get enough vitamin D are more likely to get osteoporosis and break bones. Vitamin D helps the body absorb and use calcium, which is essential for bones. When the skin gets enough sunlight, the body makes the vitamin. But between October and April in the UK, there is usually not enough sunlight for our bodies to do this. During these months, it's recommended that people take ten micrograms of vitamin D daily.

8. Eat to help your bones stay healthy

There are a lot of other essential nutrients that help keep bones healthy and strong. People should eat a healthy, well-balanced diet, says the ROS. Eating and drinking the right things can help keep your bones healthy at every age.

9. Quit or cut down on smoking and drinking

The ROS says that if you drink a lot of alcohol, you are more likely to get osteoporosis. Since smoking slows down the cells that build bone, smoking could weaken bones and make them more likely to break. But don't worry, it's not too late. If you stop smoking, the chance of breaking a bone starts returning to normal.

TAKEAWAY

Osteoporosis is a disease that can cause bad things to happen. It can cause breaks, which can hurt, take a long time to heal, and cause other problems. The good news is that there are many things you can do to both prevent and treat osteoporosis. Eat well, exercise more, and take the right medicines.

Living with Chronic Pain

TWO-FITHS OF people have chronic pain by their 40s, with consequences for later life. Chronic pain can be emotionally and physically taxing and, because it never goes away, it can make you angry and frustrated with yourself and the people around you. Whether it's an uncomfortable back, a dodgy knee, or aching joints, pain is something that every midlifer experiences.

- About 15.5 million people in the UK, or 34% of the population, have pain that doesn't go away.

- About 5.5 million people, or about 12% of the population, have high-impact chronic pain that makes it hard for them to do daily things.

- About 22% of the population, or 10 million, have low-impact, long-term pain.

- About 8 out of 10 people with chronic pain (84%) say that at least some of their pain is in their neck or shoulder, back, limbs or extremities, which are all places where the pain is most likely to be musculoskeletal (25% neck or shoulder pain, 42% back pain, and 55% pain in arms, hands, hips, legs, or feet).

Doctors often use 'chronic pain' to describe any pain that lasts three to six months or longer. The answer is not as simple as visiting the local high street pharmacy to buy pain relief pills, topical gels, or heat and cold therapy. According to NICE (The National Institute for Health and Care Excellence), there is evidence that opioids can be harmful and lead to addiction.

And if the pain is from an old injury, it can sometimes be challenging to manage pain when it comes. Runners make up the most significant percentage of athletes suffering from IT Band syndrome (80%), and sadly although I'm not a runner, I have lived with this chronic pain in my knee for years, and it has impacted how I go about my everyday life.

Aside from surgery (not an option for me), several medical procedures, such as over-the-counter or prescription drugs, can be used to manage chronic pain. They are possibilities, but focusing on your mental and emotional health is vital. I've partly developed my resilience and pain management skills because of this.

Suggestions for Managing Chronic Pain

Maintain stress control. Physical and emotional pain are tied together, and ongoing pain can increase stress levels. Learning appropriate stress management techniques like deep breathing, slowing down and taking a break will help you manage your chronic pain more successfully. You may also effectively manage your stress and pain by eating healthily, getting enough sleep, and engaging in safe physical exercise.

Be a positive influence on yourself. Thinking positively is a helpful tactic. If you focus on the improvements you are making, such as the fact that the pain is less today than it was yesterday or that you feel better than you did a week ago, your perception of your comfort level may shift. For instance, remember that even though you feel uncomfortable, you are working to discover a healthy method to handle it and live a valuable and complete life. You won't feel helpless or unable to cope with the agony if you do this.

Talk to someone. It can be challenging to deal with your discomfort daily, especially if you're doing it alone. Try to connect with those who share your experiences and can relate to your highs and lows. Look online or in your neighbourhood for support groups that ease your load by letting you know you're not alone.

There is no difference between your brain and body. Most long-term pain sufferers lose that sensation of control over their bodies. They believe they are separate from their bodies and that their bodies are mistreating them.

Exercise has been linked to a reduction in pain in 23 studies, while improving quality of life in 22 others. However, getting up and exercising can be a challenging task for someone who is in pain. If the thought of your chronic pain keeps you from going about your everyday activities – it's time to change that perception.

TAKEAWAY

There is no magic pill or intervention that makes chronic pain disappear. I have clients like myself who live with chronic pain. When you think about pain, it gets worse instead of better. Find something you like to do instead, something that will keep you busy and take your mind off the pain. You might not be able to avoid pain, but you can take charge of your life. The Midlife training programme has significantly increased pain tolerance. Participants are changing their pain tolerance by modifying their perception of pain.

Knee Pain

IN THE PAST, I have had several knee operations. But recently, one of them has been very painful; it could be age or hereditary because my mother had arthritic knees. But that has not stopped me from exercising because when you stop, the real problems start.

To many, jumping on a mini rebounder is counterintuitive to helping with knee pain. Instead, they believe jumping up and down puts too much pressure on the knee joints by squishing everything together every time you land on the mat surface. But that's not the case. I devised a gentle jumping sequence that is one of the best ways to control knee pain, stiffness and mobility and help others who also suffer from knee pain.

When someone has trouble with their knees, hips, or back, the problem may not be with the bones but with the muscles and ligaments that support them. Weaknesses and injuries can also contribute to joint pain all over the body, and pressure is the leading cause of pain. Traditional ways of working out, such as cardio with a lot of impact and lifting weights, put more pressure on these areas. They might help less than a rebounder does to strengthen the structures around the knees.

A Whole-Body Approach to Strengthening Joints

When people have pain and stiffness in their knee, they generally only think about the joint. But they should pay more attention to the muscles, tendons, and connective tissues around a joint. Jumping on a rebounder helps because it strengthens all these parts near the knees.

Over time, the structures around the knee joints lose their ability to hold on to fluid. The circulation gets worse, which makes knee pain and stiffness worse and harder to treat. Working on this area with a rebounder makes it possible to improve fluid retention and circulation in the knee joint systems.

Why Rebounding Is Better than Traditional Workouts

When joint problems start, they can quickly turn into destructive cycles that are hard to break. Because of the pain, it's harder for you to work out, so you gain weight over time. This extra weight then puts more stress on the knees and other joints, making it even harder to exercise. At some point, you may feel stuck and like they can't get better because traditional training exercises are too painful or impossible for you to do.

Rebounding is an excellent alternative to high-impact, hard exercises that can sometimes do more harm than good. Rebounding doesn't add more weight to the body, but it makes the body feel heavier by adding feelings of weightlessness and G-forces to the workout routine. Also, rebounding helps to avoid the jarring effects of regular exercise, which many people feel when they do everyday activities. Like the cycle of getting hurt, gaining weight, and having trouble working out, injuries and strain from jarring, high-impact exercises can also make it hard for someone to work out and strengthen their joints enough to feel better.

When you have knee pain, whether from an injury or being weak, it's important to strengthen all the structures around the joint that help it move. Traditional leg exercises will likely hurt you too much to get the desired results. Most leg exercises are high-impact cardio, like running and jogging, or weightlifting, like leg extensions, squats, and leg presses. When the knee is already hurt, doing hard things like these can damage it.

When you bounce on a rebounder, you can rebuild and strengthen the structures that support the knee joints. This includes the tendons, ligaments, and minor muscle groups often ignored in regular exercises. By strengthening these parts of the knees, blood flow and fluid retention are improved. This reduces joint pain and improves the way the knee joint works.

TAKEAWAY

Knee pain can be hard to treat, and it might seem silly to focus on these areas when they hurt every day from everyday things like walking and light lifting. Rebounding, on the other hand, strengthens all the structures that support the knees. As with any exercise, anyone who wants to try rebounding should talk to their doctor first to lower their risk of getting hurt.

Managing Lower Back Pain

LOW BACK PAIN is a common symptom experienced by people of all ages, although it peaks in mid-life and is more common in women than in men. In the UK, over the last 20 years there has been a 12% increase in how likely a person is to experience disability due to low back pain.

I occasionally get back pain and, like many people, short-term episodes of sciatica (four out of ten people get sciatica at some point in their lives). Mostly this will resolve itself over days or weeks without needing specific treatment but for some people it becomes chronic. Mike Tyson, the former boxer recently said that his sciatica had put him in a wheelchair and got so bad that he couldn't even talk.

The sciatic nerve is part of the spinal cord and helps move the muscles in the legs and feet. It also transmits sensations from the legs to the brain. Pain from this nerve originates in the buttocks on one side or the other and is caused by damage or irritation to the muscle structures at this level. Because of the pressure the resulting inflammation puts on the sciatic nerve, it sends pain signals to the brain. I have a sharp, 'knife-like' pain that travels the length of the leg that is affected.

Some people's pain is so bad that they can't even move. Experts at the Harvard Medical School say that about 40% of Americans will have sciatica at least once in their lifetime. The NHS says that 13% and 40% of people will have it at some point. People between 30 and 50 years old and those with acute or long-term back pain are most likely to have it.

Sciatica is often caused by a slipped or herniated disc in the spine, according to doctors at Johns Hopkins University. Discs are soft cushions with soft, jelly-like centres that sit between the bones, or vertebrae, in the spine. When these slip, the disc's jelly-like centre breaks through the lining and presses on other bones and nerves.

Our spines are unique – very complex systems of bones, ligaments, tendons, and muscles that work together to let us move in all directions. Even though all of this movement is good, it could lead to injuries and wear-and-tear damage over time, which could cause back pain and stiffness.

The most common reason motion causes back, or neck pain has little to do with the bones in your spine. Instead, it's related to the muscles and ligaments that surround your spine. You could tear one of the large muscles or ligaments that support your spine when you twist your lower back into a yoga pose or overstretch a forward fold. When this damage happens, the area around it usually gets red and swollen. This inflammation can cause a back spasm, hurting your lower back badly.

When the pain was bad, I had moments when I would have said yes to everything and paid anything to make the pain go away. But I did not; instead, opting to use exercises like Cat to Cow and deep breathing to help ease the back pain. Cat-Cow (see page 99) is an excellent exercise for the health and mobility of your spine! It's good because it's easy to do and has breath awareness. The goal of Cat-Cow is to move the spine and pelvis and change how the spine moves.

Being in pain creates bad breathing habits. But changing how you breathe can change how you feel in a big way. The first step is to pay more attention to how you usually breathe. When in pain, we often breathe in ways that aren't good for us. But with practice, changing your breathing can change how you feel. The first step is to pay more attention to how you usually breathe.

How to check your breath:

• Put one hand on your chest.

• Put the other one on your stomach, just below your ribcage.

• Rest your hands there for a few minutes while taking a few slow, deep breaths.

• Watch the hand that moves the most.

The hand on top of you moves the most: You breathe through your chest. People who are tense and in pain tend to hold their breath and only use the top part of their lungs for breathing. It's not the way to relax; it can cause muscle tension in the shoulders, neck, and chest.

The hand on your bottom moves the most: You are a diaphragm breather. This deep breathing is the best way to relieve pain and stress. Try to fill your lungs to the bottom when you deep breathe. The big muscle band under the lungs, called the diaphragm, then pushes down, which causes the belly to get bigger.

TAKEAWAY

Low back pain is a many-faceted problem that comes from your lifestyle and what's happening around you. A chiropractor, osteopath or doctor won't make your back pain disappear. You need to keep physically active in the right way, find a strategy to manage stress and keep on with normal activities.

Shoulder Pain

SHOULDER PAIN OR tightness is common; 18–26% of adults have it. Six weeks ago, when I woke up, my right shoulder hurt, not as badly as when I dislocated both shoulders years ago, but the pain is just as frustrating.

I hear a lot of people talk about how painful their shoulders are. When your shoulder hurts, you realise how important it is to your everyday movements. And that includes things like moving around in bed. Millions of people suffer health problems triggered by stress and anxiety. Could my shoulder pain be stress related?

Because it is not as protected as other joints, the shoulder joint is easily hurt. For example, the hip joint is stable because the thigh bone and pelvis fit together like a ball and socket. But the humerus, the upper arm bone, is almost too big for the shallow shoulder socket, which holds the top of the bone in place. It gives the joint much freedom of movement but little stability.

A rotator cuff is a group of muscles and tendons that wrap around the shoulder joint and stabilise the head of the upper arm bone firmly in the shallow socket of the shoulder. As the name might suggest, this helps you do a lot of different things, like holding your arm up to comb your hair or throw a ball.

The supraspinatus is the essential part of the rotator cuff. It is connected to the bone by a tendon. When this piece of tissue gets damaged, it can cause tendonitis, an inflammation of the tendon. Tendonitis can happen when you lift something heavy or when you try to break a fall. The damage could also be normal wear and tear, which happens to everyone as they age.

Once you turn 60, overusing a joint, like playing too much sport, can cause inflammation in the tendon as it tries to heal itself. As you know, the main sign of shoulder damage is pain, which is often a deep, sickening pain. The arm tells you to stop using it until it gets better.

Shoulder pain could also come from:

- Arthritis in the joint of the shoulder

- Bone spurs in the shoulder area

- Bursitis, which occurs when excess fluid builds up in a bursa, the cushioning pad between bones and tissue in joints

- Broken shoulder bone

- Dislocation of the shoulder

- Laxity in the joint space (space between shoulders), i.e. between the head of the humerus and the clavicle or scapula spur

- Frozen shoulder happens when the muscles, tendons, and ligaments inside the shoulder get stiff, making movement hard and painful

- Overuse or injury of nearby tendons, like the arm's bicep muscles

- Problems can also be caused in another part of the body, like the neck or lungs. 'Referred' is the word for this kind of pain. The shoulder usually hurts when it's at rest, but it doesn't get worse when it moves.

Here are some tips for healing shoulder pain:

If you've ever had shoulder pain after working out, use ice and ibuprofen. After 15 minutes, take the ice off and wait another 15 minutes. Do it approximately 3–4 times daily for 2–3 days. Use a towel or cloth to cover the ice. You can get frostbite if you put ice directly on your skin.

Check out this 'Floor Slide Exercise.' It stretches the muscles on the front of the body, opens the chest, and makes the shoulders less round. It works the rhomboids and lower and middle traps in the back, making them stronger. It also eases tension in the upper traps. Then when you stand up straight, your shoulder muscles and tendons stay where they should be.

- Get on the floor and bend your knees

- Tuck your chin a little, making your neck look longer

- Lower your shoulders, so they aren't touching your ears

- Raise your arms 90 degrees and put the backs of your elbows and hands against the floor

- Slowly stretch your arms out in a Y shape above your head. As you do this, ensure that your whole back, head, elbows, and hands stay in contact with the floor and that your shoulder blades stay down.

- Keep the repetitions of three sets of 10 slides slow and controlled

---

TAKEAWAY

It's essential to strengthen the shoulder joint and the muscles around it to increase its stability. More stability allows you to improve your muscles around the joint without putting that joint in a compromised position that could lead to injury. In addition to strength, it's also essential to focus on building mobility that allows you to move and control throughout a range of motion.

CHAPTER 3 – LIFESTYLE

'Set realistic expectations and goals, and be realistic about what you can and cannot do'

Body Rejuvenation

IT COMES UP behind you, but now that you're into midlife, your body changes; some of these changes are because of age. But you're not the only one who feels a bit rounder around the middle than they used to. Hormonal changes and changes in how you live can make you gain weight, especially in your 30s and 40s. And when it comes to those few extra pounds, it can be hard to lose weight.

By the time you're in midlife, you've probably reached a point where you're no longer worried about money like you were in your 20s. But some worries are just part of growing up. One of the most important is that once you hit midlife, you may start to notice that your body isn't quite the strong, high-metabolism machine it was ten years ago. As you get older, there may be times when you don't even recognise your body.

So, here's what happens to your body in midlife and sometimes what you can do about it.

People of all races and both sexes tend to get shorter over time. With age, changes in the bones, muscles, and joints are linked to height loss. After age 40, most people lose almost half an inch every ten years or about 1 centimetre. After age 70, height loss happens even more quickly. As you age, you may lose between 1 and 3 inches (2.5 to 7.5 centimetres) of height.

- *The excellent news is that you can control how fast you lose height by keeping a good posture and eating a healthy diet.*

As time passes, most people lose muscle mass, and their strength and power also go down. The process starts before you might expect. Sarcopenia, which is muscle loss caused by ageing, can start around age 35 and affects most people at a rate of 1% to 2% per year. It can speed up to 3% a year after age 60. Loss can be slight, moderate, or severe, or muscles can stay at normal levels.

- This muscle mass, strength, and function loss can be slowed with exercise and a generous amount of protein in your diet to aid muscle repair and growth.

The injuries and pulling of muscles of the midlife athlete are often more complex than younger athletes. Muscle wounds take longer to heal because hormones, biochemistry, and physiological processes work together.

- Incorporate a range of mobility and stretching exercises instead of trying to 'push through' pain or ignoring it.

Your sex drive can go down because our bodies change, and social norms tell us to slow down instead of speed up. These changes can cause problems with how we see ourselves, making men and women less sexually interested. Forty-three percent of women, and 31% of men report some degree of sexual dysfunction.

- *Men should do Kegels while making love to put off the inevitable. When you squeeze your PC muscles (pubococcygeus muscle), you tell your brain that you need to go to the bathroom, but you won't. Because your penis only has one urethra, it stops you from ejaculating. Women who do Kegels can help get more blood to their pelvic floor and vagina, which may help them get aroused and keep things smooth. During sex, a woman can also do Kegels, which can be fun for her partner.*

Some muscles that weaken the most with age are those in the urinary tract. That's why most women over menopause and men over 40 have trouble holding their urine. One study found that 68% of women between the ages of 42 and 64 had this problem.

- *Exercises for the pelvic floor muscles can help strengthen the muscles under the uterus, bladder, and bowel (large intestine). They can help both men and women who leak urine or can't control their bowel movements. One way to train your pelvic floor muscles is to pretend you have to urinate and then hold it.*

TAKEAWAY

There are more ways to age than we think. We can do something to stop or slow the process, or we can accept and live with the joint pain, tiredness, and sagging skin as they are. The question is how you want to get older. You have a choice.

Dating Minefield

ANYONE DATING AGAIN in their forties and beyond is using dating apps to try to find 'The One' while presenting themselves as a potential 'One', and knows how boring, random, and completely difficult the whole process is.

App dating isn't for everyone. We will all agree that it is a minefield at the best of times, and I can confirm that it gets even more complicated with age for both men and women. I have spent my entire life preserving and nurturing my body, so I'm in good shape. Unfortunately, most people my age cannot say the same because they have invested in different aspects of their lives. The chances of men and women like me finding someone of a similar age and ambition with a youthful attitude and lifestyle is slim.

There is no secret to a great relationship – you need to work at it. The whole thing is a numbers game for the 77% of midlife daters who have only been on between one and three dates in the past year – 63% are open to dating without commitment, and 25% are looking to get married. With maturity, you have become aware that emotional intimacy is essential in a relationship. In fact, at this point in your life, it is a prerequisite and is actively encouraged.

It leads to desperate measures on dating sites, where we downplay our age or even outright lie about it so as not to get filtered out of searches. When I talk to a potential match, I know from the first conversation if my date would be interested in dating an older man. If she is, then it is then that I reveal my actual age.

They will often ask, 'Why did you lie about your age? That's terrible.' I respond, 'Have you ever thought about a relationship with an older man before we spoke?' I believe it is more important to do what feels right with someone who makes you feel special and accept whatever the future may bring. It's a person's personality, not their specific ages, that ultimately make or break a partnership.

Perhaps naively, I have no problem with age-gap relationships because I am physically younger than my actual age and fitter than many men half my age in a shrinking candidate pool.

I no longer fear commitment, which once terrified me. I have become patient and accepting that relationships can fail or succeed, regardless of age. I know that socially a significant age gap often raises eyebrows and social disapproval, but in these enlightened times, is age an accurate reflection of who we are? Would it not be regrettable to reject someone you love because you fear what others may think? I know I'm not the only person who is young at heart, and by the same token, plenty of men and women are older than their years. Why don't we ignore the stereotypes, break the rules and shake things up a little?

Age is a number, not an assurance of health or how long you will live or that I will die sooner than you. My potential younger partners may meet someone in their age bracket, but that does not guarantee that one will not develop cancer or get run over by a car.

The probabilities of dying around the same time are more significant if you choose a partner of the same age. However, other additional factors can affect the durability of a relationship, such as the odds of both partners being faithful or the probability of remaining in love.

TAKEAWAY

Would it not be better to have loved and lost than never to have loved at all? Isn't having a life with someone you love now preferable to the risk of nothingness? Accepting who and what you are can give you the courage to live in the here and now. Follow your heart and dismiss what others think. The mind is always trying to figure out what the heart already knows.

Midlife Dressing

MIDLIFE DRESSING ISN'T to look youthful – it's to look ageless. At 58, Brad Pitt is a year older than Boris Johnson. But what they can get away with wearing is an altogether different proposition.

Yet a lack of happiness in midlife contributes to low confidence levels in how midlifers look. More than three-quarters of midlifers need to be in better shape physically, while a third admit they have never been the type to bother with doing exercise.

It's also worrying news that two-thirds of people think it's normal not to bother about their looks if they have a serious partner. And one in four people believe that keeping healthy and looking good costs too much money and is too big a commitment.

Many have 'de-tagged' pictures of themselves on Facebook because they are embarrassed about how they look in the photo. A lack of confidence in what you wear or even trying too hard means wearing clothes you regret buying. And even if you think you have a sense of personal style, only 38% of people like or wear half the clothes in their wardrobe.

Clothing choices differ between the sexes, with 40% of men wearing whatever is easy – that said, few are well-dressed. The first rule of thumb for men should be to lose your gut expansion, and you will look better immediately. You don't have to buy much from there; you can ignore trends and keep them simple. By that, I mean contemporary classics but not dull or frumpy. In contrast to men, 33% of women try too hard to fit in with trends, regardless of whether they suit them. And 48% said they regret buying items of clothes just one week after they take them home.

So, my golden rule is to find your style that fits your life and represents your best self with flair and fit. Of course, you can dress any way you like. But are you trying too hard to look young?

The best fashion statement is the real you in its healthiest state. And the key to dressing in midlife is ensuring your clothes fit right. Yes, a killer body means you can wear anything and look good, but that isn't happening for most midlifers. So, embrace your physique and age and accept the change in your body to dress in the best way possible.

Forty years ago, while in Milan, I remember seeing men and women who looked like they walked off a catwalk and wondered if I'd ever find that kind of effortless style. These days you don't need to go to places like Milan or Paris. There is a list of midlife-style icons that are tearing up the rulebook. They dress for the person they are today, not the person they were 15 years ago.

People can tell how you feel about yourself from what you wear, and it's the first thing people notice when you walk into a room. Psychologists call it 'Enclothed cognition' – how what you wear influences your behaviour, your perception of yourself, how others react to you, your confidence and your self-esteem.

My go-to casual smart uniform:

Navy Sweater

A navy sweater is the most versatile item in my wardrobe that can be matched with any article of clothing and will act as a layer in winter and a feature piece in summer.

It is also a favourite of laid-back menswear. Giorgio Armani, the 85-year-old billionaire uber-designer, said, 'The one item I can't live without? That's easy. A navy crew neck sweater, probably cashmere.' Miuccia Prada is the epitome of casual chic in her well-fitted navy sweater, knee- or calf-length A-line or printed skirt, kitten heels, and good jewellery.

White Jeans

In the summer, white jeans have a certain simplicity about them. Wearing a pair in the cold of winter is about confidence. If you think you look sharp, others will likely think so too.

Suede Chukka Boots

Chukka boots have Steve McQueen as their patron saint. They are a timeless classic that best answers the smart-casual shoe conundrum. They are the ultimate all-purpose city shoes – both elegant in style and have stood the test of time, combining comfort, function, and fashion with a classic, modest look. I'm no movie star, but I feel like one when I wear my chocolate-brown chukkas, with off-white chinos, a white T, and a blue sweater.

TAKEAWAY

There is no correct answer to the dressing in midlife question because it depends on your liking. Some may think having a stylish wardrobe is more important than having a nice body, while others may think the opposite. In the end, what matters most is what makes you feel the most confident and at ease.

Eat More Protein

THERE WAS A time when I did not eat enough protein until I learned the 50+ body processes protein less efficiently and needs more to maintain muscle mass and strength, bone health and other essential physiological functions. Yet, up to a third of 50+ adults don't eat enough.

Our bodies experience changes as we age, which we must proactively address with food. Protein will help you retain lean tissue as you age, which is crucial given that we lose approximately 5% of our muscle mass per decade after age 35. Everyone should prioritise it, including those who have never set foot in a gym.

In a 2018 study that followed over 2,900 seniors for 23 years, researchers discovered that those who consumed the most protein were 30% less likely to have functional impairment than those who consumed the least. While adequate protein intake cannot prevent age-related muscle loss, insufficient protein intake can aggravate muscle loss in older persons.

Proteins supply the building blocks for enzymes, neurotransmitters, hormones, and tissues such as muscles, tendons, internal organs, and skin. Proteins make up around 15% of the human body.

How Much Protein Do You Need?

Scientist believe we are not eating enough protein. According to Professor Stuart Phillips, an expert in muscle growth, once we hit our forties our body's ability to turn dietary protein into vital muscle starts to wither, and that we should aim for 1.6g per kilogram of bodyweight per day. Double the UK's recommended nutritional intake – about 55g on average for men and 45g for women.

Dr Oliver Witard, a senior lecturer in exercise metabolism and nutrition at King's College London, says that the current recommended protein intake will not be enough as we age. We can blame this on anabolic resistance, which gets worse as we get older. Anabolic means that it builds muscle. When we eat protein, our bodies are naturally prompted to make muscle tissue. But anabolic resistance makes it harder for the body to respond. Witard says that this starts to happen earlier than most people think, when a person is in their forties.

If 'anabolic resistance' wasn't enough to make you think about getting more protein, the word 'sarcopenia' might. This is about the loss of muscle mass and strength that comes with getting older. This can start happening as early as our thirties. If you eat enough protein, sarcopenia slows but if you start exercising in your midlife, it will help your muscles stay responsive to the protein you eat.

Does Protein Quality Matter?

Different types and quantities of amino acids are found in various protein sources. Ideally, your diet will provide a complete spectrum of amino acids. Consuming a wide variety of natural food sources, including meat, chicken, fish, seafood, eggs, and protein powder is the best method to accomplish this. The protein quality is essential, but this is only common sense. Try to eat as diversely as possible, avoid food ruts, and combine actual food with protein shakes for convenience. You will be healthy if you consume various meat, poultry, fish, seafood, eggs, dairy, grains, legumes, pulses, and beans (as your diet permits).

How to Meet Your Protein Requirements

The best approach to obtain a complete spectrum of amino acids is to consume actual food (and most animal products). However, this is not always possible, and some individuals prefer not to consume any animal protein. No matter what type of diet you follow or how busy you are, there are various tasty and enjoyable ways to maintain a healthy protein consumption.

Dietitians advise considering a protein powdered smoothie when the target is not reached through meals alone. But most protein powders are hard on the gut because they include protein sources that are hard to absorb that disrupt the delicate ecosystem that is your microbiome. For three years, I have used an organic protein powder and openly promote them. It's a plant protein with vital omegas and digestive enzymes derived from whole foods and containing a high protein concentration.

TAKEAWAY

Remember that practically all foods include protein, so consider this when determining your protein intake. The little amounts of protein in oats, potatoes, grains, and fruits and vegetables all add up. Sport, fitness, health, and nutrition are for everyone, regardless of who they are, what they do, or how they do it.

Sugar Addiction

WE ALL KNOW that sugar is not good for us, and I used to be addicted to sugar, but I quit when I realised that these sugar highs always ended with a crash, which made me want more sugar. It made it clear that I needed to make a change.

Sugar can be as addictive as cocaine, and in the same way that drug addiction happens, it triggers the 'reward centre' of the brain. When you eat sugar, your brain makes the 'feel good' hormone, dopamine. If you eat a lot of sugar, your brain will get used to the high and become less sensitive to sugar. So, your brain needs more and more sugar over time to get the same rush.

When you eat something sweet, your blood sugar increases, releasing dopamine (which makes you feel good) and insulin (which triggers your body to store the sugar as fat). Then you 'crash': your blood sugar level drops, you feel tired and hungry, and you reach for another sugary treat. The physical urges completely overpower your willpower and desire to eat well.

Sugar is in more than 70% of packaged foods and is sometimes the second or third ingredient. Think about everything from breakfast cereals to BBQ sauce, salad dressings, and so-called 'healthy snacks' like granola bars or even those 'heart-approved' refined-carb breakfast cereals.

Studies have shown that the neural chains activated by sugar are very similar to those activated by cocaine and heroin. In 2007, a team from the University of Bordeaux did an interesting experiment to determine if sugar was as addictive as cocaine.

Forty-three lab rats could choose between two 'reward levers' eight times a day for fifteen days. One lever gave them 20 seconds to drink a solution of sucrose, and the other gave them a small dose of cocaine through an IV.

In just two days, the rats made it clear that they liked the sugar solution more. They were also more likely to choose the sugar lever as time passed, even when the 'reward price' was higher (sugar came out only after multiple lever presses) and when it took longer to get the sugar. The scientist did the same experiment with a solution of saccharine, an artificial sweetener, instead of sugar, and the results were the same. It suggested that sugar addiction is caused by the taste of sweet food, not by eating glucose.

A critical part of sugar addiction is that it can cause the body to release opioid substances, the same chemicals that makeup heroin and morphine.

Studies have shown that when rodents are taken away from sugar after being used to it for a long time, they show signs of opiate withdrawal, like chattering teeth, trembling heads, and shaking paws.

Most people, unlike lab rats, can eat sugar whenever they want to, and a lot do. Making you feel hungry, you turn your attention toward high-calorie foods instead of away from them. It is why, if so many people are overweight, they keep eating more.

Food labels have over 60 different names for sugars. And be mindful that even natural sugars, like agave or honey, still contribute to your daily sugar limit. If sugar is in the top five ingredients on the label, then it's not nutritious.

And to settle the whole fruit-is-sugar debate, while fruit has sugar in the form of fructose, it's nothing compared to added sugars and doesn't cause the same blood-spiking mechanisms. There's no need to limit fruit if you're focusing on reducing added sugar.

TAKEAWAY

The simple truth is it's easier to know what's going on in your body if you control what you put into it. If you eat or drink a lot of sugary foods or drinks, that is a clear sign that you are addicted to sugar. You may always eat to avoid boredom, get too hyper, and then crash. You might even say that you want sugar after a stressful argument – this is a sign of addiction.

CHAPTER 4 – MINDFULNESS

'Take time to relax and de-stress. Practice mindfulness and gratitude and find ways to stay positive'

Midlife Transition

ARE YOU GOING through a dip in your mid-40s to early 50s? Your kids are older, your career is safe, and you're relatively happy and still reasonably healthy. So, why are you in a slump when life seems reasonable? It's a midlife transition. At this stage in life, people can start to reflect more on what their life is – compared to what it should have been. Many people thought their life would be different because their expectations of themselves were much higher when they were younger, and this can mirror their happiness level in midlife. I'm here to tell you that any negativity you may have can reverse by developing a sense of self-purpose, leading to a much more positive life after midlife.

Making myself a priority without being selfish has made me much happier. My gratitude for being fit and healthy reinforces my growing satisfaction with who I am, and this helps me to overcome any negative thoughts. I have fewer work or family issues, and a noticeable decline in stress levels has increased my happiness. I'm no longer as depression-prone as I once was. If I make a bad choice, I experience less regret than the younger me because commitment to exercise gives me the confidence to believe that things will work out – by focusing on the positive rather than the negative self.

The holistic approach of the Meta-Age philosophy involves the application of mindfulness, which provides a way to get through challenges, offering a better perspective to know that, as you get healthier, you can mentally help yourself deal with the midlife transition. We learn to accept the disappointment that our body no longer responds as it did in our twenties; we normalise it. Take this normalisation of physical change as an analogy for life; stop beating yourself up for how you feel.

Change is the only guarantee in life, and how you adapt to change will determine the person you become – negativity only worsens things. I used to be hard-wired with optimism about the future until I found myself comparing my achievements to others and believing I had fallen short. This internal criticism was a recipe for suffering. Through exercise, I began to stop comparing myself to others because I came to understand that everyone is different. Understanding my body gave me better control of my mind and stopped my inner critic from spinning out of control. My mantra became: 'I don't need to be better than anyone'.

Since midlife transition is not a disease, it doesn't have typical symptoms like a cold or flu. Here are some signs that you are going through one:

You want to know more about yourself or a particular part of your life, such as your relationships, age, or job.

You have many personal problems because you don't know who you are or your place in the world.

In the past few months, you've gone through enormous changes, like getting divorced, that have changed how you feel about yourself.

You are asking yourself important questions about your values, spirituality, beliefs, interests, or career path.

You want to give your life more purpose, meaning, or passion.

A mindful, disciplined practice can help you to turn off the self-judgment button, feel less anxious, and experience more positive emotions. It can help you become more present by switching your mood in the right direction. Spending time with like-minded people gives you the confidence and comfort to share your feelings with a cohort group that can listen without judgement and with compassion. It helps you feel that you're not alone. I've witnessed irrational behaviours whereby people try too hard to radically shake things up by throwing away their wives and family and starting over without much thought. My midlife was about progressing toward my goals – rather than achieving them – reinforcing my life of purpose to become a better person to myself and other people.

TAKEAWAY

There is no need for radical change. Incremental changes that bring small accomplishments will boost your positivity. Just because you're discontented now doesn't mean life is passing you by. Stop questioning who you are. It's what your purpose or your values are that matters. Making a midlife transition is about self-awareness and discovering your sense of self-worth.

Guide Your Mindset

SOME PEOPLE THINK meditation is weird, that it is difficult to practise, a waste of time or something that one might do when one is bored.

Everyone already practises some form of meditation. By allowing our thoughts to wander, almost sub-consciously, sifting through the chatter in our minds, while focusing on an activity – yoga, swimming, or even just walking we are practising a 'moving meditation'. Think back and ask yourself how you feel mentally after that session; I suspect many will say calmer, more clear-minded, mentally refreshed, etc. That is the fundamental aim of meditation, and its benefits can profoundly affect your mental health.

The momentum of thoughts can make us feel uncomfortable, sad or powerless about a situation, causing stress and anxiety. If we meditate regularly (e.g. a few minutes each day), we can create a new habit which will enable us to experience moments of 'non-thought' and allow a feeling of peace and relief to enter our minds.

How often have we felt disconnected, not knowing what decision to make, or making them out of need or desperation – should I take that job or not? Should I call that person or not? If we can connect to our inner self, we can achieve clarity of mind which will help us to make more positive decisions and, in turn, the desired outcomes.

Case studies have revealed that daily meditation has helped patients recover from diseases and helped them reduce pain levels.

By allowing our mind to clear from thought and releasing all kinds of physical, mental and emotional resistance, we are allowing our cells to do what they do best: recover and heal themselves.

In our quiet moments of reflection, inspirations come flooding in. The influx of ideas or moments of inspiration can be encouraged by engaging in tasks and living in the moment, allowing creative thoughts to flow and time disappears.

For people suffering from chronic stress and depression, quieting the mind can be challenging. Moreover, people can be scared of going inside their minds as they do not feel they have control over their thoughts and will end up in a 'bad place'.

With meditation, we can create a new habit allowing us to recognise when uncomfortable thoughts are starting to creep in. Once we realise that we can control our mind and how it works, we will feel empowered and confident in our capacity to find peace of mind, no matter what.

We are constantly bombarded with signals, disinformation, and ideas, and, for some people, there is no relief – day or night. When we reach a saturation point, we can no longer cope logically or calmly when a stressful situation comes our way.

Sleep is a great way to re-boot the mind, but for some people, this is not enough since as we dream, we might retain the vibration of our problems and have stressful dreams or even nightmares. By releasing our conscious thoughts through meditation, we allow our mind to free itself.

It is hard to recognise when negative thoughts overtake us, when we reach saturation point, or have extraordinary stress factors, but it can all build, gaining force and volume, becoming more of a threat as it grows.

Meditating, especially at the beginning of the day, can halt that slow build of negative thoughts, prevent the 'snowballing', allow us to feel more secure and connected, and shift into more positive thinking.

TAKEAWAY

The art of meditation is a very personal journey. The method, meaning and results are different for each one of us. We are all wired differently; our minds are the best reflection of this. The way we see the world and how we process information is unique to each one of us. The most important thing is to start meditating and watch how your life changes for the better as you learn to mind your mindset.

Moving Meditation

HYPNOSIS AND MEDITATION both have the potential to induce altered states of awareness. One can become calm and focused by being guided or persuaded, without taking medicines. Practitioners generally use hypnosis to help people stop bad habits, whereas meditation focuses attention and raises awareness.

KUN-AQUA meditative walking has the potential to do both and bring physical benefits by using the sensations of water as your focus as you try to keep your body steady like the mast of a ship against the movement of the water.

The difference between sitting meditation and KUN-AQUA meditative walking is you keep your eyes open. That difference implies other changes in the way you do the practice. You are not withdrawing your attention from the outside world like when you are doing other mindfulness breathing practices. You are aware of things outside of yourself that you will be more aware of than when you are sitting – especially if you sit inside. But one of the most significant differences is that it's easier to be more aware of your body in water when compared to sitting forms of practice.

When your body is in motion, it is generally easier to be aware of it compared to when you are sitting still. Sitting still in meditation, the sensations that arise in the body are much more subtle and harder to pay attention to than those that occur while you move, making KUN-AQUA walking meditation an intense experience.

KUN-AQUA walking transforms itself into an intense spiritual practice as you aim to walk without effort. There is mindfulness in that you must align your belief in what you think with your actions of what you do. You are bringing yourself in touch with all the wonders of life within and around you. Walking this way is the appearance of non-exercise – the attainment of non-attainment.

Walking in water slows not only our movement but also our thinking process. It helps us understand the interconnectedness of our bodies and minds to help achieve effortless pleasure in what we do.

Don't try to control your breathing. Allow your lungs as much time and air as needed. With each step, you fully align yourself, posture, balance and focus before making the next step. When you're sure you've arrived in the here and the now, feeling the body aligned, you make the next step. Walking like this, you develop stability, awareness, and strength in the water. The key is mindfulness.

During walking meditation, we walk relaxed, with a light smile. When we practise this way, we feel deeply at ease, and our steps are those of a secure person. Water walking meditation is really to enjoy the walking, walking not to arrive, just for walking, to be in the present moment, and to enjoy each step. Therefore, you must shake off all worries and anxieties, not thinking of the future, nor the past, just enjoying the present moment. Anyone can do it. It takes only a little time and a little mindfulness.

KUN-AQUA meditative walking has enormous positive effects on longevity and general health. It is an exercise practice with considerable positive outcomes and almost mystical heart-building, fat-burning, and life-enhancing properties.

The amount of exertion used positively affects the metabolism, improving blood sugar levels and reducing insulin resistance because of the effect on our powerhouse cells –mitochondria. These cells are essential in creating energy to drive cellular function and all biological processes. They make your body better at converting fuel into energy to make you stronger and healthier. Also, the mitochondrial decline in older individuals is likely an outcome of decreased activity levels rather than ageing.

Walking in water provides many benefits and burns fat as fuel rather than carbohydrates. It is a discipline where your body is working, but not overly hard-working, to about 60-70% of your maximum heart rate, where you should be able to hold a fully realised conversation.

Each session takes enough time for you to remain entirely in control of your exertion. At the same time, you provide a meditative approach to enlist a different mindset to the usual goal-focused determination of gym exercising.

TAKEAWAY

Meditation is typically associated with stillness, lying or sitting in a comfortable posture with a focus on the breath. Yet, movement can also provide a path to contemplation. Stepping through water from one foot to another can be a moving meditation. The practice of yoga, qigong, tai chi and aikido also form the foundation for moving meditation.

'When our mind is not happy and balanced,
it leads to tension in the body, which manifests as the
potential for disease'

Resilience and Stress

I LEARNT A long time ago that stress, in some form, will always be a part of my life. It's an unavoidable challenge that has wreaked havoc on my body and mind in the past.

So how do I protect my health from the effects of stress when I know it's a fact of life? I learnt the hard way that I could not change the stressful event, but I could build resilience. When a stressful situation happens, over time this resilience has lessened the impact of stress and how I feel about the situation. A recent study suggests that a lack of resiliency to stress is the reason stress is harmful to your health, not the stress itself.

What is Resilience to Stress?

Think about the last time you were stressed about something. Maybe an argument at home. Were you able to shake it off quickly, or did you dwell on it for hours or even days?

Your ability to quickly bounce back to your usual self after a stressful event is called resilience. Fixating what causes stress, and letting it spiral into deeper negative emotions causes a single stressful moment to have a ripple effect, leading to chronic stress and a potential impact on mental and physical health.

Why Resilience Matters

A recent study published in *Psychological Science* suggests that your level of resilience can determine whether stress will cause long-term harm. The study surveyed more than 1,000 adults about daily stressors (such as at work, home, or school). Then, the scientists asked them how long the stressors typically affected their mood.

Almost ten years later, the scientists surveyed the same people again. They asked them about their physical health, chronic illnesses, and how much they felt their health interfered with day-to-day activities. This was to evaluate how stress resilience affected a person's health.

The scientists noticed a fascinating relationship between persistent stress and health effects, noting, *'Higher levels of lingering negative affect are associated with greater numbers of chronic conditions and worse functional limitations ten years later'*.

This suggests that those who dwell on stress are significantly more at risk of developing health issues. Although small amounts of stress are expected, it's your body's response to an immediate threat: a release of adrenaline that provides the boost of strength and speed you need in order to react quickly.

Some amounts of stress are good to push you to the level of optimal alertness, behavioural, and cognitive performance. But when stress becomes chronic; when the stressor or pressure is persistent and affects you over a long time, it becomes a problem.

How Resilience Works

Let's say you get out of your car and spill your smoothie over the passenger's seat. You have two choices: let what happened hang like a dark cloud, or you can take deep breaths and tell yourself, 'Well, shit happens!', clean it up and get on with the rest of your day.

Getting stressed usually doesn't help, but acknowledging your feelings and then releasing them so you can move past them is an example of strong resilience.

Resilience is what keeps short-term stress from becoming chronic and harmful. It's the path that will lead you to greater happiness and improved emotional health.

Ways to Improve Resilience

Of course, you can't just snap your fingers and magically develop it. It's a skill that needs to be practised. There are some simple tricks you can use to build or improve your resilience. Work on shifting your perspective on life and practise the following three tips:

1. Daily Meditation

Meditation helps to improve your control over your own emotions. It lets you be in control of your feelings, dictating how you react to the world. Everyone has time to meditate; even a few minutes can help calm the mind. By focusing on being present, stresses can melt away.

2. Focus on the Good

Bad things happen, but so do good things. When dealing with something stressful, think of the good things in your life. Practising gratitude, even for small things, will help shift your perspective and focus on something hopeful.

3. Take Deep Breaths

The next time you notice yourself getting stressed, step back and take eight deep breaths. It will allow you to keep a level head in a stressful situation so your emotions don't rule.

TAKEAWAY

Resilience is the inner strength you can draw on to bounce back from stressful things – it is the missing puzzle piece in managing stress. With greater resilience, you will learn how to be happier and thrive so that nothing can hold you back.

Sound Confident

IF YOU WANT to sound like a person who is sure of themselves, you have to change your whole way of thinking. You must appreciate that to sound confident you must also listen and give others the tools they need to grow.

Be Yourself

Talk in a calm, soft voice. Don't try to be too loud and sound like a strict teacher. Use the words you usually would. Use formal language sparingly because it will make you sound and feel stiff.

Try this exercise before you speak to calm your voice:

1. Face a wall and stand there.

2. Put both hands on the wall at about shoulder height and push hard, like you're trying to move the wall a couple of metres in the direction you're going.

3. After pushing, stand up normally and try to speak out loud.

Hear how much calmer and more connected to your feelings your voice sounds.

Be Present

Be spontaneous. If you stay in the moment, the people you are talking to will do the same.

Start Well

Try to get your main point across in the first sentence so that people immediately pay attention. 'That shirt/dress looks great' could be a great conversation starter. Practise saying your words out loud and give yourself time to practice. One hundred and fifty words per minute is a good rule of thumb.

Talk with Energy, Clarity, and Kindness

To speak excitedly, you use about 10% more energy than usual which can make you sound like the host of a game show if you use too much power. You must be clear in what you say and how you say it. Most importantly, you need to talk in a way that shows you care. It's the way you speak and the words you choose that make you interesting and believable.

Try this simple trick to sound calm and in touch with your feelings. If you're standing, squeeze your buttocks or thighs for ten seconds, then slowly release. It will make you and your voice sound calmer. And no one will be able to see you do it!

Don't Make Everything about You

Always try to sound like you are equal to the person you are talking to but make sure your main focus is about them. Remember that it's not about you. They say 'Pride goes before a fall'. People will want you to fall on that banana peel if you look too good.

Don't Think of the Audience as a Single Big Group

When speaking to a group, it's easy to 'lose focus.' The key is making eye contact and to appear to convey one thought with one person and another thought with another, so that everyone feels like you're talking to them.

Don't Avoid Awkwardness in the Room

If you think someone isn't on your side and is holding on to prejudices or fears, it's usually best to talk to them about it instead of trying to hide or avoid it. Unless you do this, they won't pay attention to what you are saying.

Don't Take Yourself too Seriously

When we see someone taking themselves too seriously, we can't wait for them to spill their coffee or trip over a loose cable. A little humour that pokes fun at yourself goes a long way.

Don't Rush

Wait two seconds before you say something. If you start talking too quickly, it will sound like you want to get the conversation over as quickly as possible. So, stand and wait for two seconds before you speak. It will make it look like you are comfortable where you are and give you a natural air of authority that will impress people.

Doing this simple breathing exercise before you talk is a great way to slow down:

- Slowly breathe in through your nose for three counts.
- Slowly breathe out for three counts.
- Repeat three times.

The whole thing should take 18 seconds. In that time, you'll be able to slow down your heart rate and feel better.

TAKEAWAY

To sound confident, we need three main things: energy, clarity, and humility. If we show all three, we'll come across as authentic, humble, and charismatic.

Are you Anxious?

ANXIETY IS A common but complicated problem that affects almost everyone at some point.

When anxiety hits, what happens to the body? How do you ride a roller coaster? How can things get better over time?

When anxiety strikes me, there is panic and a rush of fear. It is made worse by these and other scary feelings, but they don't help in any way. Often, the physical symptoms that come with the first feelings of unease can lead to a full-blown panic attack. So, what's happening inside of me?

I learned that even though it might not feel like it, the body responds in a very complex way. Dopamine, serotonin, and adrenaline help us deal with real or imagined fear. Our heart rate increases, we breathe faster, and we might get palpitations, sweat, stomach pain, a headache, or lose our appetite. It can make us tired, restless, and hurt our muscles.

Also, long-term conditions like insomnia, digestive problems, chronic pain, depression, and drug abuse are all linked to anxiety. Anxiety can also signify something wrong, like diabetes, thyroid disease, or heart disease.

What to Do if You Have a Panic Attack

According to the NHS website, you shouldn't let your fear of panic attacks run your life.

Because panic attacks always go away on their own, the symptoms don't mean anything wrong will happen. It would help if you told yourself that your anxiety causes your symptoms.

- Do not look for things to do.

- Hold out until it's over.

- Do your best to keep going.

What works for me might not work for you, but I try to stay in the

situation until the anxiety disappears. I do my best to face fear head-on and not to run away from it. It's only then that, more often than not, I discover nothing terrible will happen. And, as the anxiety starts to fade, I become more aware of what's happening around me and keep doing what I was doing before.

Exercises for Breathing During Panic Attacks

During a panic attack, if you're breathing quickly, a breathing exercise can help you feel better. Try this: focus on nothing else as you breathe in for a count of five and out for a count of five. Stay focused even if your mind is racing. In a few minutes, you should start to feel better. You might feel worn out.

- Do breathing exercises every day to help prevent panic attacks and ease them when they happen.

- Do regular exercise, especially aerobic exercise, to help you manage stress, release tension, improve your mood, and boost your confidence.

- Eat regular meals to keep your blood sugar stable.

- Avoid caffeine, alcohol, and smoking, which can worsen panic attacks.

- Join a panic support group to learn how to deal with your attacks.

- Try cognitive behavioural therapy (CBT) to find and change negative thought patterns that worsen your panic attacks. Your doctor can put you in touch with groups in your area.

Regular exercise is an essential strategy. It doesn't have to be complicated; even a quick walk can get enough chemicals in your brain to make you feel better and get your mind off things. If you don't already, try to find at least 15 minutes a day of bouncing to get your heart rate up.

It's also a good idea to try mindfulness, which almost everyone knows about, but only some of us do right. In its simplest form, mindfulness is staying in the present. If you focus on your body's sensations, feelings, and thoughts (rather than the content of your thoughts), your head may stop racing, and your stomach may stop churning. Mindfulness takes practice to become a natural way of thinking and acting, but the effects will be clear from the start.

Build a network with friends and allies. It is also essential. If you want to talk about your anxiety, you might find joining an anxiety support group helpful. Identification has a lot of power and will lead to solutions. You could also join a volunteer group in your area. You might not have time to save the world. Still, volunteering groups tend to attract friendly, helpful, and knowledgeable people who are the perfect antidote to all that thinking and imagining in a new setting.

TAKEAWAY

What enabled me to take control of my anxiety was to change my lifestyle, and I know that this method has helped others too. But if that does not work, there is medicine to help you get your anxiety under control. Think about using the Samaritans. They offer phone help 24 hours a day, seven days a week.

CHAPTER 5 – TRAINING

'Fitness is more than just working out. It's about finding balance in your life and making time for yourself'

Fitness – It's an Age Thing

MIDLIFERS NEED A rethink about their fitness and lifestyle. What's needed is a self-purpose and an entirely fresh approach for a completely different life stage. To extend midlife and reverse the typical ageing phenomena of muscle loss and cognitive change, to achieve and maintain healthy body weight, composition, and mental acuity.

At my gym, I see people putting pressure on themselves to exercise more, train harder and perform at their peak to lose weight. What they really need to do is re-evaluate their mentality.

There is a difference between feeling a burn when performing squats and experiencing pain in your hips or knees as you age. The distinction between pain and soreness is threatening to your body.

For every age group, exercise has an essential social and fitness aspect. The 45-plus age group know that getting their body into shape in 'midlife' is a different challenge from the one they faced at 20. My training methodology is the first-of-its-kind programme dedicated to training the midlife body. It is an intelligent mix of ancient and new practices involving no jogging, sit-ups, or weightlifting.

It is a programme created explicitly for age-related change, empowering positive ageing, fitness, and longevity. Every 45-plus gym-goer wants to be biologically and physically younger than their biological age, able to live a longer, healthier life. Otherwise, what is the point of exercising?

Ageing is a natural and inevitable process, but how we age is different for everyone. A growing body of research supports the immediate benefits of exercise and meditation and how they might preserve and protect our physical body and brain structure to extend our golden years and shine even more brightly in old age.

In their 20s, people take their bodies for granted. In their 30s, they start to know their body better and what it is capable of. In their 40s, gravity, hormones, slowing metabolism, decreased lean muscle mass, and increased body fat starts to creep in. That is the time to begin re-wiring the body.

Midlife Fitness at 45-plus

The training is no more complicated than traditional training, but it is more innovative and effective. The exercises alleviate age-related symptoms, increase metabolism and testosterone and improve mobility, flexibility, and endurance. Training in the right gym environment can also benefit mental and emotional well-being.

It combines two unique mind and body programmes, JUMPGA and KUN-AQUA, created explicitly for mid-lifers, which are better than any drug a doctor could ever prescribe. Their goal is to achieve peak mind and body performance for the 45-plus body to combat age-related change.

The two programmes comprise compound movements incorporating upper and lower body strength training and core exercises. All the moves are low impact, and the easy-to-follow workouts combine all six components of optimum fitness:

- cardiovascular endurance
- muscular endurance
- muscular strength
- flexibility
- body composition
- mobility.

Older gym-goers can be divided into three groups: those who have never stopped exercising, those who have lapsed, and those who have never trained. These two programmes will encourage all three groups to get into or continue training – and have fun along the way.

After 30, your body can lose 5% of muscle mass every decade. A study published in *The New England Journal of Medicine* found that, with proper exercise, older people can avoid muscle weakness and frailty.

Fit midlifers don't categorise themselves by age but by who and where they are now, and it's exhilarating to know they have 20 to 30 years of prime living to do. Society would have them believe this time is the beginning of the end.

My training facilitates the continuation – or return – to flowing, unimpeded movement without being unduly conscious of physical ability. It serves as an essential guide in the process of behavioural change. Both JUMPGA and KUN-AQUA advocate mindful movement and self-control through pranayama. It starkly contrasts many popular fitness activities (including yoga) that can have an aggressive approach, often leading to muscle strain, joint pain, ligament tears, or just a negative exercise experience.

These encounters or injuries can, in turn, cause emotional distress, depression, and anxiety, which are primary triggers for weight gain and ageing – the very things midlifers are battling against when they exercise!

KUN-AQUA

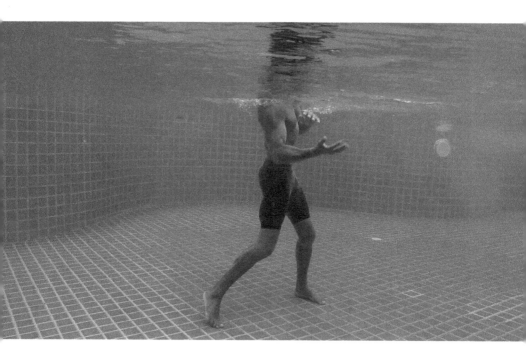

KUN-AQUA PRACTICES date back thousands of years, emphasising intense mind and body control. Mindful practices melded with water resistance exercises to form a mind and body experience that can enable people to regain control of their bodies after years of neglect; for young aspirational yogis and gym-goers looking for an alternative, lower impact form of exercise; for captains of the industry keeping themselves fit and healthy, as well as their businesses; and for sportspeople looking for that extra edge to get them over that last hurdle and to their ultimate goal.

KUN-AQUA: Training but Better

Practitioners have said that they experience a meditative state of mind during KUN-AQUA. This can happen in many forms of exercise when we control our breath to create more energy in our bodies.

KUN-AQUA emphasises doing only a few simple movements to bring awareness into how and what people do, as this is far more important than rushing through a series of exercises without any presence. On a yoga mat, one-leg balances are often the most challenging exercise of yoga, and the act of trying to maintain balance and achieve the pose takes the focus away from breath control and good posture. Doing the same exercise in water allows people to concentrate on rooting down the base leg and focusing more on posture because buoyancy takes the weight off the joints. Once your awareness is on the standing leg, you can initiate deep diaphragmatic breaths and work on the alignment of the body up from that base. The muscle memory process translates directly to improved stability on the yoga mat on dry land.

'Water training is the ultimate resistance exercise.' ## The Mayo Clinic

A person's ability to balance remains functional until around 40 but gradually declines. If they don't have core strength or mobility through each joint to perform an exercise safely, their body is at risk of injury. This is because proper form involves moving through a range of movements consistent with the function of the joints involved. Underwater training is slowed by water resistance, forcing practitioners to flex and extend the joints more slowly than they would on land, enabling them to work on maintaining proper body positioning and focus more on correct form – far more important than how many repetitions they perform.

There Are Two KUN-AQUA Programmes:

KUN-AQUA Meditative Walking improves self-esteem and confidence, and encourages relaxation. There is a sense of accomplishment as you master how to do it. In many religious traditions, walking forms a spiritual bridge between meditation and everyday life. Mindful walking is meditation in action. Like anything else, walking can be done either mindlessly or mindfully. It's too easy to be mindless and drift away with thoughts and fantasies whilst living on autopilot. Gaining the full benefits from meditative walking requires conscious control of the breath; to control prana and thus to control the mind, the key to realising all the benefits of any asana.

KUN-AQUA Athletic is a total body workout. It recruits muscle fibres from every angle and therefore requires incredible activation and stabilisation of all the muscles. It can burn 30% more calories than by practising the same workout on land. It is not 'Aqua aerobics', where people jump around breathlessly; all KUN-AQUA movements are about proper form, moving the body in a controlled manner through a complete range of motion. Unlike regular weight resistance training, where there is momentum and gravity to assist, in the water, the resistance is the same at the beginning, middle and end of the movement. The heart must also work harder to provide blood to the muscles, resulting in improved cardiovascular fitness.

KUN-AQUA Training Facts

Over 50% of body weight is water, but this is effectively reduced by as much as 90% when standing in water up to neck level. Yet water provides 12 to 20 times more resistance than air, making it the perfect place to get fit. Working out in the water activates muscles from every angle, building overall strength faster and increasing muscle definition while putting minimal load through the joints, thus significantly reducing any risk of injury.

KUN-AQUA burns about 30% more calories than the equivalent exercise on land. The extra water resistance makes the heart, lungs and muscles work significantly harder, which can result in rapid increases in strength and stamina and decreases in body fat content.

Water has the added benefit of hydrating, oxygenating and revitalising the body's musculoskeletal system. The effect of gravitational pull is removed, and weightlessness qualities are achieved. A whole range of exercises, including intervals, stretches and balances become more sustainable, resulting in increased endurance.

Hydrostatic pressure – or the pressure in water at rest due to the weight of the water above that point – causes the heart to pump more vigorously. This can lead to better lymphatic drainage (decreasing swelling in the joints and soft tissues) and a reduction in blood pressure.

Hydrostatic pressure also supports the joints, improving their alignment without exerting any stress. It becomes easier to move joints through their full range of motion and reach full extension and flexion. This leads to greater flexibility and improved proprioception (body awareness).

Water training disperses body heat about four times faster than air at the same temperature, naturally helping to maintain the core body temperature within an acceptable range and preventing the overheating common with vigorous, land-based exercise.

'Lèal has left me with a fresh definition.
of fitness and the fight against age.'
Phil Hilton, *The Times*

JUMPGA

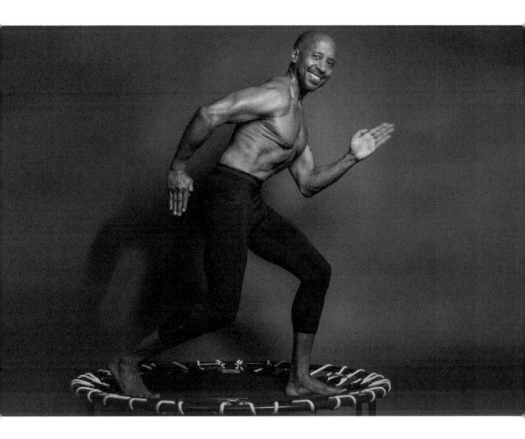

JUMPGA, the yoga fitness hybrid, is endorsed by Yoga Alliance Professionals. It incorporates two disciplines: rebounding and yoga. It is the perfect re-introduction to exercise as the rebounder floor constantly moves – challenging all the core, stabilising muscles, and the body's centre of balance most safely and uniquely. It's a holistic lifestyle programme for people who want to future-proof their bodies as early as possible. It introduces yoga asana to the most resistant people, including professional boxers and footballers.

'It's a great workout for balance, cardio & strength.'
Sun newspaper

Using the rebounder as a prop during yoga sequences enables a person to feel the benefits of the postures regardless of their level of flexibility, age or physical condition. It can help them access postures they might not otherwise be able to do. It will help modify the poses as they learn the fundamentals of yoga. Placing their hand on the rebounder to stretch into poses can help them to lengthen their spine safely. Similarly, lying on the rebounder can strengthen their lumbar spine in poses like Bridge.

'JUMPGA the new yoga and trampolining hybrid – might be the one for you' Madeleine Howell, *Telegraph* newspaper

It was the yoga master Iyengar's ingenious use of props that helped practitioners at all levels to gain the sensitivity of a pose and receive the benefits over time, but without over-extending themselves. Students could practise the poses and breath control with greater effectiveness, ease, and stability. It is a yoga asana for the 'average' person. Keeping the yoga asana element simple makes it easier to perform the postures, no matter how inflexible or unfit people think they are.

JUMPGA will be the most potent form of movement: a complete holistic cycle – from ecstatic jumping to the peaceful meditative state of savasana. Physically, it produces molecular changes in muscles, like going for a long run and lifting weights. Thus, it provides the same fitness benefits as prolonged endurance training but in much less time.

When the then 31-year-old former middle-weight boxing champion of the world, Darren Barker, discovered the root problem of his debilitating injuries was because his fitness training exposed his body to more force than it could withstand, he turned to JUMPGA. The outcome was a 14-week injury- and pain-free training camp that culminated in him becoming the first man in modern boxing to become a world champion without running, skipping, lifting weights or doing a single sit-up.

The Benefits of JUMPGA
- Metabolic rate – the metabolic rate increase can last up to 24 hours. During this time, the body continues the accelerated breakdown of sugars and fats, processing oxygen and building muscle.

- Weight loss – the excellent news for calorie counters is that rebounding puts the numbers on their side. Someone weighing 75 kilos who goes for a 30-minute jog expends energy equal to about

175 calories. The exact time spent doing JUMPGA cardio burns 205 calories, and it's way more fun!

- Circulatory system – jumping on a rebounder increases heart rate, oxygen uptake and efficiency of the lymphatic drainage system.

- The focus on breathing (Pranayama) boosts physical and mental well-being. It becomes a whole-body workout that strengthens the heart and lungs and increases the immune system.

- Muscles – exercising on a rebounder works all of the muscle groups. Just steady bouncing for a few minutes can lead to an improved sense of well-being, or push fitness levels through the roof with the JUMPGA sequence of yoga asanas, plyometrics and callisthenics, making it the best comprehensive training programme.

- Flexibility – jumping on a rebounder strengthens, lengthens and tones muscles all at the same time.

- Bone density – exercise can strengthen bone density as well as muscles. Increased bone density helps to prevent broken or fractured bones and the onset of osteoporosis.

- Joint, tendon and ligament function – the strengthening of joints, tendons and ligaments can help to reduce the chances of some forms of arthritis and lessen the pain in some arthritic joints.

- Balance and coordination – balancing on a rebounder is unlike balancing on anything else. The rebounder floor is constantly moving, so it uniquely challenges all the core stabilising muscles and the body's centre of balance.

How often should you jump? Every day is best. Doing a gentle bounce for 5 minutes in the morning can help you wake up and prepare your body for the day. That's enough to get your lymphatic system and blood moving, so is an excellent way to start. Build up to HIIT training: Jump as fast as you can for 30 to 60 seconds, then rest until you fully recover. Do this again and again for 15 to 20 minutes. It is a great way to get your body to burn fat for the next 24 to 48 hours.

'Try Yoga on a Rebounder especially if you are over 40'
Madeleine Howell, *Daily Telegraph*

HIIT

MODERN LIFE HAS people feeling time-poor and pressured to find the most efficient ways of using their time when they're not sleeping. Hence the fitness regimen of high-intensity interval training, or HIIT.

HIIT is an interval-based workout combining short bursts of intense exercise with periods of rest or lower-intensity exercise. I taught my first interval-based programme over 40 years ago, but HIIT didn't hit the mainstream until about a decade ago when exercise physiologists demonstrated that intervals could deliver the most noticeable health improvement within a short amount of exercise time. An article in the *New York Times* in 2013 popularised HIIT with a seven-minute workout and, since then, scientists have looked beyond the surface and discovered proven benefits that elevate HIIT beyond a way to lose weight.

Here are five basic questions about HIIT answered.

1) First things first: What is HIIT?

HIIT workouts generally combine short bursts of intense exercise with periods of rest or lower-intensity exercise. They mix aerobic and resistance training.

When researchers talk about HIIT, they're referring to workouts that alternate hard-charging intervals, during which a person's heart rate reaches at least 80% of its maximum capacity for one to five minutes, with periods of rest or less intense exercise.

2) What does a HIIT routine look like?

What differentiates HIIT from the steady-state, continuous types of exercise – jogging at an even pace or walking, for example – is the intervals, those periods of heart-pounding intensity. If you want to try it, you can take a HIIT class, run, or even walk in a way that involves higher-speed and higher-incline bursts.

A Norwegian lab-tested routine involves a warm-up, followed by four 4-minute intervals (again, where your heart rate reaches past 80% of its maximum capacity), each interspersed with a 3-minute recovery period, finishing with a cool-down.

For instance, you might jog for 10 minutes to warm up, followed by four intervals of faster running lasting 4 minutes each, split with a 3-minute interval of moderate jogging, and an overall cool-down of 5 minutes. It should take 40 minutes to complete the process.

Alternatively, the 10-by-1 interval regimen consists of 10 1-minute bursts of activity separated by 1 minute of recovery; a more condensed but well-researched form of an interval workout. I allow 45 seconds of recovery.

3) What advantages does interval training offer?

Improved heart health is the most well-established benefit of interval training and has been scientifically proven. A study from 2016 tracked the VO2 max of two participating groups over 12 weeks. VO2 max has been shown by research to provide a good general health indicator and is an endurance test to measure the amount of oxygen the body can take in. The better your heart can pump blood, the longer it takes you to exhaust yourself, and the farther and faster you can ride a bike, run or swim, the more aerobically fit you are.

In the study, one group exercised for 10 minutes (including a series of 1-minute intervals), while the other for 50 minutes (at a continuous pace).

The study's most striking conclusion was that, despite having different time commitments, both groups of exercisers had an improvement in their oxygen uptake. Interval routines lead to more significant gains in VO2 max compared with other forms of training in a shorter time. HIIT is a time-efficient strategy to get the benefits typically associated with more prolonged bouts of traditional cardio.

I have long used the interval technique to help athletes up their game. They mimic their 3-minute rounds by doing four to five times of 3–5-minute intervals.

4) Why does HIIT improve cardio health?

Researchers say it depends on the heart's ability to pump blood. One measure is the volume of blood that comes out when the heart contracts, and a significant determinant of VO2 max is stroke volume. The maximum amount of blood from the heart can be improved by interval exercise training, and the stroke volume increases even more.

5) Is HIIT the best exercise regimen for weight loss?

There's no doubt that interval training can be a time-efficient way to burn calories. Consider a longer interval routine if your goal is weight loss. Add some continuous steady-state training to have a higher resting metabolism and to burn the fuel in your body quickly.

But it is still easier to lose weight by cutting calories in your diet than trying to burn excess calories.

TAKEAWAY

Researchers at the Charles Perkins Centre at the University of Sydney found that three to four short bouts of exercise like HIIT showed a 40% lower chance of dying early. When you do HIIT regularly, your aerobic fitness gets much better in a short amount of time. It's a programme for people who want an easy way to change their eating and exercise habits and get healthier.

Super 6: Exercises

YOU DON'T NEED a gym to get fit or stay in shape, and using your body weight is one of the most effective strategies to increase your strength and fitness.

Doing these Super 6 exercises engages more muscles simultaneously than if you were using weights, where you tend to isolate the effort to one body region. When we utilise our bodies instead of machines, we enhance core use and use our stabilising muscles more, which are essential for everyday movement and injury prevention.

What results from stringing together these six exercises, health bounce, single leg stand, squats, and push-ups, bird dog, and Cat-Cow regularly? You receive an excellent full-body workout with or without the need for equipment.

Daily reinforcement of the benefits of exercising can lead to long-term changes in behaviour. New psychological research involving the University of Warwick, concluded that simple repetition is the key to hacking the brain to form solid habits. Can it work with helping develop an intrinsic motivation to exercise? Yes, it can.

My training principles align with the research. Working with professional athletes, I witnessed how habits result from what they desired versus what they did. I'm not a psychologist, but desire plays a big part in motivating our behaviour.

These six simple exercises build discipline, self-confidence, and focused awareness.

There are three essential components: the goal, learning the exercises and reinforcing self-confidence. Providing goals instils the ability to take responsibility for your actions and learning.

This will help you to:

- foster a 'can-do' attitude

- establish discipline and intrinsic motivation

- encourage the setting of personal objectives

- instil pride in overcoming difficulty.

Getting fit is specific, measurable, and trackable. How many press-ups, squats or star jumps can you do in one minute? Every exercise provides an incremental objective that can help you stay motivated, continue to improve and achieve your personal best.

The absolute beauty of Super 6 is its simplicity. Six simple exercises turn fitness from extrinsic to intrinsic motivation for life and build self-confidence that promotes well-being. It is challenging yet achievable and will help you understand how to develop and thrive in life.

I use a rebounder to make the movements more of a challenge and reduce stress on the joints, but the outcome is me being twice as strong. And so should you, so you can feel movement sensitivity as you access those hidden sensations inside you.

Health Bounce

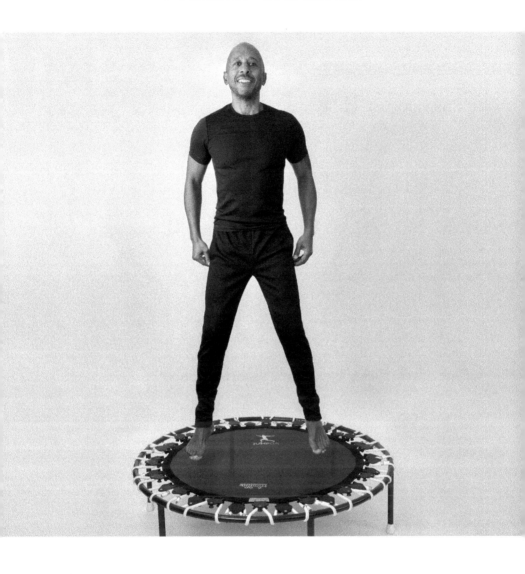

Many health and physical practitioners will use elements of a simple five S.T.E.P.S. approach (Stretch, Therapy, Exercise, Posture and Strengthening), which empowers back-pain sufferers to manage pain themselves without the need for painkillers.

The Health Bounce can be done on the floor but is best carried out on a rebounder. It offsets hours of sitting and can be applied to your lifestyle and exercise regimes, but, most of all, during your working day.

Each time you land, focus on pressing down instead of jumping up. Not every move starts in the middle of the mat and ends there. How well you can control your bounce and how central your feet are on the mat are more important than how high you jump.

When you are doing the health bounce on a rebounder it is important to:

- Try always to be aware of where your body is while on the rebounder. You can do this by working out in front of a mirror or looking down at your feet every so often, to ensure you're in the centre of the mat.

- Keep a 10–15-degree bend in the hips, a slight bend in the knees, and proper alignment through the feet, knees, hips, spine, and neck.

- Don't bounce too high or out of control (your feet shouldn't leave the mat by more than two inches)

- Remember that bouncing with narrow feet requires more control than bouncing with wider feet.

- Keep your core engaged and your eyes fixed on something still across the room to help you to stay stable.

There are three types of Health Bounce:

One: Feet wide: bouncing on the mat with both feet.

Two: Raise and lower each heel while keeping the toes on the mat.

Three: Take your feet about 1 to 2 inches off the rebounder in a small jump.

How does Health Bounce help you?

You build key muscles with every jump, improving your balance, strength, and heart health.

The Health Bounce combines vertical jumping to strengthen muscles all over the body with a low-impact landing because the rebounder cushions the landing much better than solid ground. It works quickly, is strong, and is easy to do. When you bounce or jump, your heart rate also increases, which is good for cardiovascular health.

What makes up Health Bounce?

Several movements make up the bounce, each working different muscles.

Hip extension

Imagine you are sitting in a chair and then getting up. A hip extension is what you do when you want to get up from sitting. The first part of the jump happens before your feet leave the mat or ground. It primarily works on the muscles in the upper leg, like the gluteus maximus and adductor magnus. Every time you jump, you use these muscles and strengthen how they work.

Knee extension

The knee extension straightens the leg at the knee joint. It is done almost at the same time as the hip extension. Most of the work for extending the knee is done by the quadriceps.

Ankle plantar-flexion

As you jump, Pointing your toes is the last thing you do with your body before your feet leave the mat. It is the plantar-flexion of the ankle, which is done mainly by the calf muscle.

Shoulder abduction and flexion

Jumping is an excellent exercise for the lower body that can be done independently. Moving your arms while you bounce can make it even more of a workout.

Squat Strength

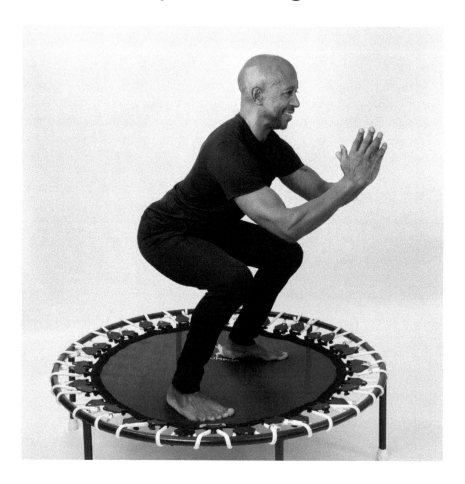

THE SQUAT EXERCISE engages all the major muscle groups, improves fitness, and helps build strength. It can increase blood flow to the pelvic region, boost libido, make orgasms more intense, and enhance athleticism in the bed or on any playing field.

There is a lot of debate about the best way to do a squat. I can only speak from experience about the safest way to benefit from this compound movement.

The lower you squat, the more your spine becomes a limiting factor that often leaves you limping out of the gym. Better to be safe than sorry and do a half squat to keep your spine safe and build strength where you need it. Only a tiny proportion of people who exercise can execute the full squat safely and effectively. Most people give up because of back tension – not because their legs tire. So, unless you can isolate the movement into the hip and lower limb, you will cause compression on your lumbar spine and can end up with blown discs.

Key Points

1. Squatting strengthens the core. Apart from the leg muscles, the core must work hard to maintain excellent posture during the squat. You can expect to make faster improvements, perform better at other exercises, and lower the chance of injury and postural difficulties if you have a strong core.

2. Because the squat is a compound exercise, it engages several muscle groups. The gluteus maximus, gluteus medius, quadriceps, hamstrings, hip adductors and abductors, the core and abdominals, and several other smaller muscle groups are used to complete the squat exercise.

3. Strength in the leg muscle groups means that the joints in and around your legs are safer when performing everyday tasks like stair climbing, walking, running, sitting, and standing.

4. Squats build lower-body strength and size. While isolation exercises on machines are fantastic for targeting muscles and increasing size, the squat's ability to demand participation from many muscle groups leads to faster total muscular growth in less time and, again, in functional strength.

During mid-life, your tendons, muscles, and ligaments become less elastic. The squat is an excellent exercise, stretching and strengthening the muscles, tendons and ligaments surrounding the leg bones while you exercise and increasing your muscle mass. Also, squats burn calories and are arguably the best strength exercise you can do anywhere, reducing the likelihood of knee and ankle injuries.

How to:

1. Stand with your feet about shoulder-width apart and slightly turned outward (about 5 to 7 degrees for most people during a bodyweight squat).

2. Make an arch in your foot by pressing down on your heel, the base of your first toe, and the base of your fifth toe to make a tripod. It will help you stay stable and spread your weight evenly.

3. Drive your hips back into a hip hinge, bringing your chest forward and working your glutes and hamstrings.

4. Squeeze your glutes and push your knees out to make your hips tight and turn outward. You should feel your outer hips contracting. It helps you keep your form safely, protecting your knees and back as you go deeper into the squat. Make sure to keep the arch in your feet and keep all three points of the feet on the ground.

5. Make sure your neck and torso are straight and neutral. Look straight ahead and a little bit down.

6. Go down to the position you want, parallel to the ground or above. Stay balanced by spreading your weight evenly between your feet.

7. Drive your hips up and back and pull your shins in until they are vertical as you stand back up (the ascent).

Single Leg-Stand

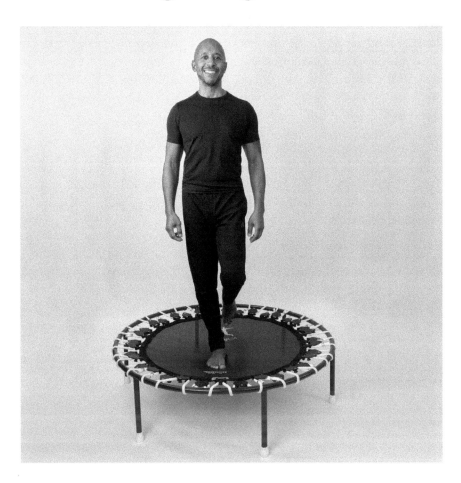

A HEALTHY WORK-LIFE balance means different things to each of us but achieving it is a realistic objective. My emphasis is on a balanced body whereby each part of the body works with another so that the body is balanced.

Workplace and home stressors are frequently to blame for our lack of work-life balance. However, studies' results explain why exercise is so beneficial in achieving a better work-life balance: people who exercise regularly have a higher sense of self-efficacy.

Physical balance aids in preventing falls, whereas mental balance aids in the prioritisation of tasks. It is something that most of us intuitively grasp. We don't realise how vital physical balance is and how exercising our physical balance may help us enhance our mental health.

As a martial artist, you stand in position knowing you're stable and safe and, at that moment, your personal confidence grows. Feeling shaky or unsteady has the opposite effect, making confidence feel as rickety as a structure built on shaky ground. The more balanced you can stand, the more self-assured you become, and this will quickly spread to other areas of life.

Physical balance is a skill that you can improve with effort rather than it being an inborn trait. Learning a single leg balance on a rebounder is challenging. Still, with repetition over time, the confidence you gain from improving your balance will have a significant positive impact on your mental health.

The capacity to properly focus can feel like a superpower in today's distracting environment. There are numerous strategies to improve focus, including those on this list. Still, it's difficult to concentrate when you're feeling unsteady or concerned about something most people take for granted, such as the ability to stand or move without falling.

Improving your physical balance might help you concentrate better. You'll notice that your focus improves when you're not distracted or concerned about maintaining your balance.

The Good Stuff

The routine is best performed in front of a mirror to maintain good form. Athletes without injury have found that this routine helps to prevent muscle and joint damage and improves performance.

Step-by-Step Instructions

1. Stand with feet parallel, hip-distance apart. Shift your weight to your right leg, so the left foot is lightly touching the floor. Either extend your arms for balance or keep them at your sides. Look straight ahead, roll your shoulder blades back and down, and make your back straight.

2. Raise the left foot off the mat. Maintain your body position – shoulders, chest open, back straight, and head and neck in a neutral position aligned with your spine.

3. When you can comfortably accomplish (2), repeat the same sequence and slowly lift your straight arms in front of you to shoulder height. Inhale slowly and deeply as you raise your arms, exhale slowly and deeply as you lower your arms to your sides again. Repeat five times.

4. When you can do (3), try the same sequences with your eyes closed.

How long should you be able to balance standing on a solid floor?

The following numbers were taken from studying different age groups who balanced on one leg to find a normal range.

• People under 40 with eyes open averaged 45 seconds. With eyes closed: 15 seconds

• Those aged 40-49 with eyes open averaged 42 seconds. With eyes closed: 13 seconds

• People under 40 with eyes open averaged 45 seconds. With eyes closed: 15 seconds.

• Those aged 40-49 with eyes open averaged 42 seconds. With eyes closed: 13 seconds.

Push-Ups

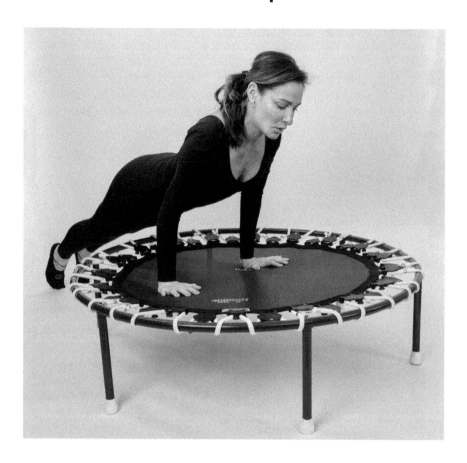

DID YOU KNOW that push-ups are said to be the best sign of cardio-vascular health and longevity for males? Over ten years, researchers collected data from 1,104 male firefighters in a study on cardiovascular (heart) disease. They discovered that males who could do 40 or more push-ups had a 96% lower risk of heart disease than guys who could do only ten. They are also the cornerstone of the fitness world and are a go-to exercise for fitness experts worldwide.

I have over forty years of fitness experience, and I still witness how push-ups instil fear in most people. Some people associate push-ups with intimidating fitness regimens or being used as a punishment. I understand this fear because I have witnessed a gym teacher, sports coach, and martial arts instructor use push-ups for failure at some tasks.

Push-ups are far more than a simple upper-body workout. They develop the core muscles while working the pectorals, deltoids, and triceps. Push-ups increase general fitness and health by increasing muscular endurance and lean muscle mass and improve upper body definition.

Push-Ups vs Bench Press

According to researchers, push-ups activate the abdominal muscles 51% more than bench press repetitions with parallel weight. It demonstrates why push-ups are the best functional exercise for training muscles to do everyday activities safely and efficiently - because they involve the integration of limb and core muscles.

Push-ups on your toes, without a doubt, are the most effective since they require more activation in the muscles of the upper body and core, as well as whole-body integration. However, doing push-ups on your toes can be difficult, and many people, especially older people or those who are new to fitness, cannot do repeated push-ups on their toes safely. The hips and neck are out of alignment, and the risk of injury outweighs the benefits. You should not quit or become disheartened if you have difficulty lowering yourself to the ground in a toe push-up position. Kneeling push-ups are an effective adjustment and because the muscle activation in knee and toe push-ups is the same, you'll quickly be able to do push-ups on your toes. Either way, there is no excuse to leave this key exercise out of your training.

The Most Effective Push-Up Technique

Here are the four crucial things to remember if you want to accomplish great push-ups:

• Spread your hands wider than your shoulders.

• Take a deep inhale as you lower your chest down to elbow level.

• Move the body as one strong body unit

• Squeeze your glutes and brace your core.

• Exhale as you push up.

Bird Dog

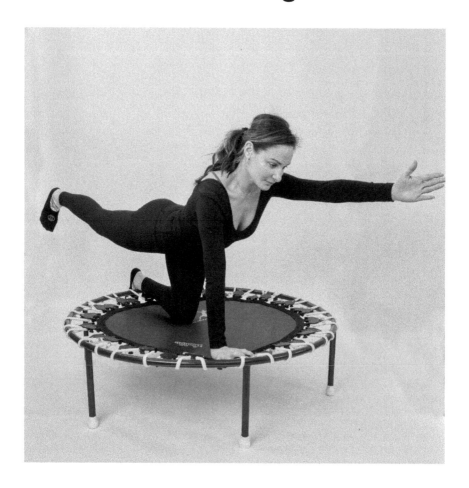

BIRD DOG IS a bodyweight exercise that strengthens the trunk muscles – more specifically, the abdominal muscles, lower back, butt, and thighs. It is also known as the quadruped exercise. It can easily be integrated into any trunk training routine. I do it on a rebounder because it is comfortable on my knees, and it makes the exercise much more challenging.

Benefits of Bird Dog

1. Bird dog can increase your core stability. Bird dog builds trunk strength and stabilisation by activating abdominal muscles including the rectus abdominis and obliques.

2. Bird dog can improve your posture. With proper form, the bird

dog exercise can strengthen your back muscles such as the erector spinae. This will help with maintaining a good posture, whatever you are doing.

3. Bird dog can enhance your mobility. The bird dog puts all four of your limbs through a nearly full range of motion, activating muscles like the deltoids and triceps in your upper body and the glutes and hamstrings in your lower body. With practice, bird dogs strengthen the muscles around your joints, improving mobility in your arms and legs.

The erector spinàe muscle is the main target of the bird dog – the long back muscle that runs from the skull, neck, and ribs down to the vertebrae and sacrum of the hip. It is in charge of moving the spine forward, backwards, and turning.

Bird dog exercises work the rectus abdominis and the obliques, two essential abdominal muscles. The move also uses the gluteus maximus muscle in the buttocks, the trapezius muscle in the upper back, and the deltoids in the shoulder (when raising the arm). It engages both the trunk and back muscles at the same time, which is suitable for building low back strength.

The erector spinae muscle is the main target of the bird dog – the long back muscle that runs from the skull, neck, and ribs down to the vertebrae and sacrum of the hip. It is in charge of moving the spine forward, backwards, and turning.

Bird dog exercises work the rectus abdominis and the obliques, two essential abdominal muscles. The move also uses the gluteus maximus muscle in the buttocks, the trapezius muscle in the upper back, and the deltoids in the shoulder (when raising the arm). It engages both the trunk and back muscles at the same time, which is suitable for building low back strength.

Step-by-Step Bird Dog

Start by doing 2–3 sets of 6–10 reps on each side. Choose your repetitions based on how well you can keep your form throughout them.

1. Start on all fours, with your knees bent and your toes touching the floor. Your knees should be in front of your hips, with your hands right under your shoulders.

2. With both hands still on the ground and turn your shoulders out to work your lats. Your ribs should be down, and the pelvis tucked in a little.

3. Ensure your shoulders and hips are tight and engage your trunk. Your chin should stay tucked like you were trying to hold an egg under your chin.

4. Keep your balance as you stretch your right hand forward and push your left heel backwards, with your toes pointing to the floor.

5. Your shoulders and hips should be parallel to the floor, and your pelvis should stay still. You should have an extended right arm and a long left leg.

6. Pause for a few seconds with your right arm and left leg extended, then slowly move back to the starting position and switch sides.

Cat-Cow

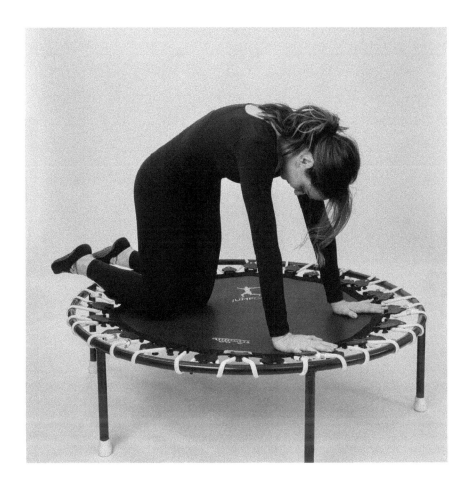

THE BEST WAY to make your spine feel better is to train your muscles, ligaments, tendons, and bones to move together in a coordinated way.

Loading the spine in weird positions, such as when doing sit-ups, is the worst thing you can do for your spine. Instead, you can improve the optimal movement when training in disciplines such as KUN-AQUA, JUMPGA, and balancing exercises.

During a Cat-Cow flow, our spine gets what it needs. It's getting oxygenated blood flow and moving through its normal and complete ranges of motion. Our spine bends and straightens, which helps develop and strengthen its primary and secondary curves (sacral, lumbar, thoracic, and cervical). This process also creates space between the vertebrae, which could help with back pain and sciatica.

All of this puts our spines in a state of balance and rest. When this happens, our brain gets the message to be calm and peaceful. So, even though our spine is the primary beneficiary here, it's clear that the benefits go far beyond that.

Advantages of Cat-Cow

Cat-Cow is a slow flow between two poses that warms the body and makes the spine more flexible. It stretches the back and neck and gently stimulates and strengthens the organs in the abdomen. It also opens the chest, which makes it easier to take slow, deep breaths. The kidneys and adrenal glands are stimulated by the movement of the spine in the two poses. Coordinating this movement with your breathing can relieve stress and calm the mind.

This sequence also helps the body become more aware of its posture and more balanced. It puts the spine in the right place and, if done regularly, can help prevent back pain.

Cautions

People who have hurt their necks should keep their heads in line with their torsos and not tilt it forward or back. If you're pregnant or have a back injury, you should only do cow pose then bring your spine back to its neutral position. Keep your belly muscles working throughout this exercise to avoid any strain in your lower back. Always work within your limitations and skills. Talk to your doctor before doing yoga if you have any health concerns.

Instructions

Start on your hands and knees with your wrists under your shoulders and your knees under your hips. You should point your fingertips to the top of your mat. Put your knees and shins about hip-width apart. Put your head in the middle and look down with a soft gaze.

1. Move into cow pose by inhaling as you lower your belly towards the mat. Lift your chin and chest, and look up towards the ceiling.

2. Widen the space between your shoulder blades and pull your shoulders away from your ears.

3. Next, move into cat pose: As you exhale, pull your belly button towards your spine and round your back towards the ceiling. This pose should look like a cat stretching its back.

4. Don't force your chin to your chest, but let the top of your head drop towards the floor.

5. Inhale as you move back into cow pose, then exhale when you move back into cat pose.

6. Repeat 5–20 times, and then rest by sitting back on your heels with your torso straight.

Doing Cat-Cow can warm up the body and prepare it for many different activities. When practising this sequence, keep the following in mind:

- Let your head fall back and relax the back of your neck to play cat. Do not force your chin into your chest.

- Also, when you do cat, you can improve the abdominal massage and strengthening by pulling your belly button firmly towards your spine.

- In cow, the movement should begin at the tailbone. Allow your neck and head to be the last part of the movement.

- Keep your shoulder blades broad and move your shoulders away from your ears. It helps to keep your neck safe while you move.

- Be aware of your breath and how it fits with what you're doing. As you inhale and exhale, picture your breath going up and down your spine, like a wave coming onto the beach and returning to sea.

TAKEAWAY

As with both JUMPGA and KUN-AQUA, The Super 6 exercises advocate mindful movement and self-control through pranayama (breathing). This is in stark contrast to many popular fitness activities (including yoga) that can have an aggressive approach, often leading to muscle strain, joint pain, ligament tears, or just a negative exercise experience. These encounters or injuries can, in turn, cause emotional distress, depression, and anxiety, which are primary triggers for weight gain and ageing – the very things midlifers are battling against when they exercise!

EPILOGUE

Thank you for taking the time to read my book. I have
slowed the decline of my ageing with intelligent choices.
I have shared insights about my lifestyle with you
so that you can all live healthier, longer and look
better doing it!

It is my firm belief that fitness is a social responsibility.
We have it within each of us to slow the ageing process,
but only a tiny percentage of the population achieves
this goal. Maybe you will be one of those too.

Wayne Lèal

Ingram Content Group UK Ltd.
Milton Keynes UK
UKHW020355040523
421174UK00010B/119